CW00521981

HIPPOCRATES
OF LONDON

HIPPOCRATES OF LONDON
by
Docteur Cybirdy

Foreword by
Dr Robin Lawrence MA
MRCP MRCPsych

First published in paperback special edition, 2022
By Cybirdy Publishing Company
101 Camley Street, London NIC 4DU

CYBIRDY
Publishing Limited

This book is sold subject to the condition that it shall not, by way of trade, digitalisation or otherwise, be lent, resold, hired out or otherwise circulated without the publisher's prior consent in any form of binding or cover other than that in which it is published and without a similar condition being imposed on the subsequent purchaser.

Docteur Cybirdy has asserted her right to be identified as the author of this work in accordance with the Copyright, Designs and Patents Act 1988

Designed by Kaarin Wall & Docteur Cybirdy
Photographer Zolo Sokob
Cartoonist Frits Holtz
Proof-read by Afaf Shour
Printed by Swallowtail Print, Norwich

This book is typeset in Minion Pro
A CIP record for this book is available from the British Library

ISBN: 978-1-7396637-0-4

DISCLAIMER
This is a work of fiction based on true events. Colleagues, patients and friends have been anonymised in this book by changing their names. Real stories are told in respect of the universal Do No Harm principle and the UK GMC good doctor guidelines

FRONT COVER
Main image: © Stuart Cox / Victoria and Albert Museum, London
Other images: iStock.com – kool99 / Neustockimages / AYImages

Page 100: gettyimages.co.uk – zahoor salmi

HIPPOCRATES OF LONDON

DOCTEUR CYBIRDY

CYBIRDY
Publishing Limited

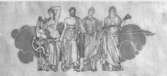

HIPPOCRATIC OATH

I SWEAR by Apollo the physician and Asclepius and Hygieia and Panacea, invoking all the gods and goddesses to be my witnesses, that I will fulfil this Oath and this written covenant to the best of my powers and of my judgment. I will look upon him who shall have taught me this art even as on mine own parents; I will share with him my substance, and supply his necessities if he be in need; I will regard his offspring even as my own brethren, and will teach them this art, if they desire to learn it, without fee or covenant.

I WILL IMPART it by precept, by lecture and by all other manner of teaching, not only to my own sons but also to the sons of him who has taught me, and to disciples bound by covenant and oath according to the law of the physicians but to none other.

THE REGIMEN I adopt shall be for the benefit of the patients to the best of my power and judgment, not for their injury or for any wrongful purpose. I will not give a deadly drug to any one, though it be asked of me, nor will I lead the way in such counsel; and likewise I will not give a woman a pessary to procure abortion. But I will keep my life and my art in purity and holiness. I will not use the knife, not even, verily, on sufferers from stone, but I will give place to such as are craftsmen therein.

WHATSOEVER HOUSE I enter, I will enter for the benefit of the sick, refraining from all voluntary wrongdoing and corruption, especially seduction of male or female, bond or free.

WHATSOEVER THINGS I see or hear concerning the life of men, in my attendance on the sick or even apart from my attendance, which ought not to be blabbed abroad, I will keep silence on them, counting such things to be as religious secrets.

IF I FULFIL this oath and confound it not, be it mine to enjoy life and art alike, with good repute among all men for all time to come; but may the contrary befall me if I transgress and violate my oath.

Foreword

The Hippocratic oath has united the medical profession for many centuries, and almost every generation of doctors from all over the world either swore this oath or something like it upon qualification.

Certainly, Dr E and I from different countries and in different languages swore by Apollo (and various other Greek gods) to uphold a medical ethic approximately 2,400 years old at the very start of our medical careers. From GPs to the super specialist doctors of every hue made this commitment. Any oath that has born such an enormous test of time, place and person deserves to be given great respect. Here, Dr E, a colleague and a friend, has demonstrated its current relevance by a series of brave, honest and revealing autobiographical episodes taken from her lifetime of medical practice.

I have known Dr E for more than twenty years. We have referred patients to each other. Members of my family have become her patients. Even as she has carefully hidden her true identity, we can all experience her emphatic commitment to the oath. A delight for me to learn more of her backstory, but an illuminating and fascinating collection of cautionary tales for every interested reader.

The oath covers areas as diverse as taking detailed notes, to confidentiality, to teaching other doctors. Holistic approach to illness is recommended but the most memorable phrase from the Oath is, "First do no harm."

Hippocrates, a physician from Kos, around 400 BC, had such an enormous impact because of the reassurance this oath gave to the patients. An Apothecary or a Physician knew about the strong potions that could be derived from plants, tree bark, seeds and berries. They knew how these could be used as poisons as how they could be used to heal. Therefore, before Hippocrates, his oath and his medical school, when a doctor was called to your home by your family you had no way of knowing whether they had come to poison you or to heal you.

These early doctors had the power of life and death; they were being paid by family (or husband) who may or may not have had your best interests at heart. Hippocrates stated that a physician should never use his art to the detriment of the patient, therefore, a doctor bound by the oath was safe. As an aging member of a large family with a fever, if a doctor were to be called, the only wise choice was a doctor who had sworn the Hippocratic oath. Any other doctor may bring poison in his bag in order to send the aging relative on their way prematurely rather than any healing balms. This reason, more than any other, caused the enormous impact of the Hippocratic oath on the practice of medicine from then to the present day. Unsurprisingly, Dr E, with her lifelong respect for an oath she took over thirty years ago, comes down strongly against doctor assisted suicide.

When E qualified, the Hippocratic oath was not controversial. Indeed, it was seen as the basis of all medical practice. All tenets are illustrated from Dr E's more than thirty years of practice. From her earliest days as a young locum GP in the French countryside, through the Aids epidemic, to the present.

The reader will be surprised upon how many fronts the modern ethical doctor has to fight. Subtle changes are shown for what they are. Dr E's commitment to traditional, ethical, medical practice shines through. Her current practice is built upon the double foundation of philosophy and experience. Both are revealed in this honest, fascinating account of her medical career.

Dr Robin Lawrence MA
MRCP MRCPsych

Wherever the art of medicine is loved,
there is also love of humanity

HIPPOCRATES

Prologue

It happened like many times before.

She is sitting in her home on the red velvet sofa. She looks up to see a long corridor; she stands and walks through. The corridor is filled with rooms. All doors are open. As she walks by, she observes. Each room has a colour theme: indigo, vermillion red, and various yellows. The indigo room contains a beautiful carpet and a Louis XV console table, the vermillion red room is filled with oriental cushions and a deep green ottoman. The mellow yellow space is occupied with opalescent art nouveau furniture with light coming through to fill the room. She does not enter. She keeps walking through. And then, she sees him.

Hippocrates sits on a great, white throne, holding his kithara vertically on his left thigh. She knows him but she does not say his name. His eyes meet hers slowly, and their metallic blue transparency makes her feel like she might be looking at herself. His body sits immobile and upright; his posture is statuesque. His face, neck and uncovered right shoulder resemble porcelain while the rest of his body is draped with a long, immaculate himation. Hippocrates' hands are ever so slightly moving. She watches the subtle shift of his fingers on the chords: his thumb is turned upward, and he plucks one string while the other fingers are held horizontally, slightly curved. They stare at one another. She does not feel fear. She stays and watches him until he opens his mouth and says with the voice and the words of her mother, "The future belongs to the early birds." She wakes up.

Dr. Elpis smiled at her dream. She rose from her bed and let the voice of her mother ring in her ear. She remembered that phrase well, it was one of her mother's many idioms. *L'avenir appartient à ceux qui se lèvent tôt.* 'The future belongs to the early birds,' she remembers the woman used to address her every morning with those words when she would join her in the kitchen before breakfast time.

Elpis was always the first of her siblings to wake up. The little girl's voyage of discovery would begin as soon as she woke. First, she stayed close to her mother and observed her morning routine. She watched the woman's hands move as they prepared the food. They were hard working hands, with damaged skin insulted again and again by the elements: fire, water, wax, paint and even bleach. The skin was dry, nearly callous, and ingrained with dirt and walnut paint around the cuticles of her short cut nails. Her mother's hands were agile though, they had been guided and protected by the repetitive skills and common sense she'd learned at a young age. Her mother did not speak much, only when necessary and often used idioms to make her point. 'The future belongs to the early birds', was one of them.

As a young child, Elpis seldom travelled beyond her Breton village and the grey granite church. It was her beacon for whenever she got lost, a piece of art she could always refer to. The church was quite stunning, made to impress young minds, like it did to the primitive pagans of the Middle Ages in Brittany. The gargoyles were apocalyptic dragons, and there was a famous statue of the pagan messenger of death called the *ankou*, sharing a wall with Christian artefacts.

Elpis left Brittany at eighteen. She went to Paris to study medicine and, following her graduation, returned close to her family. A few years later, she moved again, this time to London to learn about nutrition at the School of Hygiene and Tropical Medicine near Russell Square in Bloomsbury. And as it so often goes in life, she stayed much longer than she originally intended and settled in the megalopolis.

As a doctor trained in the eighties, she respected and revered Hippocrates. The myth surrounding him was a kind of nomism she applied to classic culture and respect of traditions that was central to her doctoring.

She pledged the Hippocratic oath on the day of graduation and never ceased to be guided by it.

For the past thirty years, the doctor had watched as anomie

became more and more settled within society. She watched as people struggled to find the possibility of a happy future. As a doctor, she looked after people within society, and as anomie was developing, she had to adapt and change the way she could treat and connect with her patients. People were lost. Sadness was spreading in this new, unhealthy environment where basic human laws of respect and care were shrinking in concert, day by day, like a skin of sorrows.

The doctor never stopped hoping though. Her connection with Hippocrates and his teaching was intense. This helped her to keep going and hoping. However, Elpis needed something else and that was to help others to regain hope.

In 2018, she made a crucial decision.

She would pass on what she knew to help the younger generation to escape the inevitable road that the world was paving, a road that was disconnected and uncaring. She would tell her own experiences of being guided by the Hippocratic oath, the universal and intemporal ethical guide. She would pass the message on actively. She knew it could never be forgotten.

Once she decided on her destiny, she felt the urgency to seek solace in the wisdom she bestowed and transfer it. It was like an act of mind letting. She had to become a mind donor. But how? The doctor was stuck until one moment of serendipity. One day, while she was googling, she came across a blog with an astonishing title, 'The Anthropology of the Native Digitals.' Not only was the title wicked, what was written was nearly extraordinary.

The author, a girl named Melo, was writing simple accounts of what she saw, heard, and even smelled, while studying groups of people within their environment. The authenticity was transpiring. There were no opinions or analysis on this blog, just raw material of the human experience reported with intelligence on topics ranging from the cultural melting pot to Japanese art and coworking modalities in London. The writer even called upon Socratic philosophy on a few occasions. Anomie was described as a fear these young people were struggling with, a fear without a name. Melo was using clever references; the writer was a wunderkind. It was obvious that Melo was a digital native too, she must have been born after the early nineties. This was what Dr. Elpis needed.

She carried on reading her essays with enthusiasm, being carried by the joy of discovering new ways of life. One essay caught her interest: it was about a coworking office in London and was documenting how young people from different backgrounds with different projects organised their days together in every innovative way. What Elpis liked about Melo's writing was that it was an objective description of human life in a particular context. It was a non-judgmental science.

The evidence was there in front of her eyes. Melo Smith seemed like the sign that she'd been waiting for. She would be the one who could listen and write about what the doctor had to say. Elpis typed a message.

"Dear Melo,

My name is Dr. Elpis. I have been a Harley Street doctor for many years. I am writing to you because I am searching for a voice. I found your blog, and I think that you might be the person I am looking for. I need someone with your talent and reputation to document my stories. Anonymity and authenticity are both essential to my project. If you want to know more, meet me at The Mirage restaurant in Soho this Saturday morning at 7 am."

▲

Melo was preparing for her usual pre-dinner meeting with her father, checking emails and messages and logging off for the day when she got Dr. Elpis' message. She was amused by it. But didn't feel the need to address the ominous request just yet. She closed her laptop, then made her way down the stairs to her father's library.

Outside the library, she saw that the door was left open. This was the agreed upon signal between father and daughter. If the door was open, she could enter. If it was closed, she could not. She pushed the opened door and entered the space as usual.

The library was a multifunctional living space linked to the man's intellectual life. It was like one of those workshop spaces of a goldsmith before industrialisation, or even a present-day artist's studio. Everything was by some magic at the right place, at the right time. As a linguist by profession, Melo's father lived among books. His library was characterised by a mix of British and French cosiness with a warm, velvety, classic indoor space, where books and their readers were kings of the show.

Her father was sitting on the velvet sofa getting ready to smoke his pipe. The moment was a ritual for father and daughter. Melo crossed the room quietly, as the man was filling his pipe bowl with a loose pinch of tobacco, pressing it down gently with the tamper. Melo joined and sat down in the corner of the sofa, bringing her legs up and tightly to her chest. Her father carried on with a few test puffs, and then lit the flame to the pipe bowl in a circular motion, drawing on the pipe all the while.

"How has your day been?" the father began.

"Good, I went to the educational seminar I told you about last week. Not many people attended though, it was a bit boring. On Tuesday, I played with the band in the studio, it was good. I got a strange message today."

"From where?"

"A Harley Street doctor that likes my blog, she's asked me to meet her for a potential project together."

"And?"

"The doctor did not give any more information, she just proposed to meet."

"Should you ask more?"

There were a few minutes of stillness. The father drew two puffs and moved closer to his child, instinctually putting his arm over Melo's shoulder.

"Did the Doctor give you a name?"

"Elpis."

"Elpis, hope after disasters. The pandora box myth, you remember."

"I do remember … I think I'm going to go."

"I think you should too."

And so it was decided. The following Saturday morning, Melo would meet Dr. Elpis at The Mirage.

▲

The young blogger took the underground from Richmond to Oxford Circus, the shopping epicentre of London. She'd never travelled there alone before. Her mother offered to drive her, but her father had replied that the journey would be easier by underground on a Saturday morning; and besides, Melo was perfectly capable of traveling on her own.

As she walked up the underground escalator, she let her eyes roll over the scene around her: it was quiet, not many were awake yet in London, only working men and women, and the athletic types. As she came to street level, Melo crossed diagonally over Oxford Circus.

She hadn't been in this part of the city since she was a child, but she remembered it well. It was the first place her father brought her to explain the feeling of *omoiyari*, the sense of others, and respect for each one. When she was a girl of just eight years old, her father placed her in the centre of Oxford Circus and she felt part of the people moving in so many different directions. It was not scary to be in the middle of the crowd, just enjoyable.

Today, she walked all alone with her head down—her blonde curls billowing in the wind—as she yearned for that feeling. There was no *omoiyari*, yet she enjoyed the lonely journey to The Mirage and wondered what would wait for her. Who could this Dr. Elpis be? And so, she walked on with that curiosity leading her forward. To her surprise, she saw a homeless man sleeping and dreaming on the pavement. She left a tenner in one of the little boxes, careful not to wake the sleeper, who had a smile on his face.

A moment later, she arrived at the entrance of The Mirage. She opened the door to what seemed like an empty restaurant. She entered and was welcomed by a kind, pretty waitress with blue eyes, a small pert nose, and dark hair. She looked like Mia Wallace's double from Pulp Fiction.

"Melo, I presume. The doctor is waiting for you. I'll take you to the back."

Melo followed the Mia look-alike to the dark, isolated back of the restaurant. The Mirage was filled with brick walls and small candles; the light seemed to have been set for secret conversations and rendezvous. As they turned a corner, someone in a hoodie—a woman—sat at a wood table with a cappuccino in front of her.

As Melo approached, the hooded individual stayed seated. She didn't raise her head to look at her, but simply said, "Good morning. Thank you for coming. Do take a seat, please." Her voice was artificial and disconnected. It dawned on Melo that her host's voice was being distorted by something. She sounded robotic and unnatural. On the side of her right cheek, Melo noticed a small lavaliere mic hooked over her ear. She assumed the doctor must be using this to transform her voice. The stranger's hood was covering three quarters of her face. She didn't move; she remained silent with her head down. The cappuccino had not yet been touched.

Melo sat as she and the waitress waited and watched the hooded individual silently. The atmosphere was strange, almost eerie. Still, Melo felt welcome by the faceless woman. She was intrigued; she'd been told from the beginning that anonymity was essential, but a meeting with a hooded figure was not what she had expected.

The waitress finally broke in. "What would you like to drink?"

"A green tea will be fine," Melo replied. "Have you got matcha tea?"

"I'll bring it straight away." And the waitress left, leaving Melo and the hooded figure alone.

"Melo, I am pleased you have decided to come. Allow me to introduce myself. I am Dr. Elpis, and I am the messenger."

Melo felt unease at the ambiguous, almost mocking response from the computerised voice, but chose not to interrupt.

"I've read many of your blog posts on the digital world and the millennials you are addressing as digital natives."

"Thank you for taking the time to read my work. I feel it's my life's purpose to reflect on my generation and what we must change for those that come after us." Melo took a moment to take in the situation at hand. "Dr. Elpis, why am I here?"

"You have a lot of followers," Dr. Elpis replied. "Your blog has gone viral. You know that."

"I guess people are looking for another narrative."

"That's exactly what I'm looking for," the doctor replied.

The matcha tea was served.

"You know, Dr. Elpis, I went into anthropology because I like to observe people, and anthropology is about people. There are no assumptions, classifications, or statistics, I don't turn people into numbers. I look and write about them as the complex individuals that they are. I've watched how people my age have deteriorated and are suffering because of digital advancements. We are disconnected, and I write to try to convince people to go back to our roots, to their culture." Melo took a moment.

"Doctor, why am I here?"

"I need to connect with a younger mind. My profession is at risk because it has lost its founding beliefs. I have carried stories with me all my life, but do not have the practice to share them with the world. You and your blog do. This is about narrative, narrative of the past, present and future, it is about morals and renewal, and I know that a few can help the world get there. We just need to connect."

"What did you have in mind?"

"I suggest that we arrange twelve meetings on consecutive Saturdays. Same place, same time. Each time, I will tell you a story to illustrate one particular moral issue mentioned in the Hippocratic oath."

"What is the Hippocratic oath?"

"The oath is the text that began clinical medicine. In most universities, it is still customary for graduates to pledge the oath to remind and uphold medical standards and ethics. However, the message has been lost, in a metaphorical sense. It is my purpose and hope to bring about a kind of resurgence."

The doctor went on. "The oath, created in the fifth century before Christ, was written by Hippocrates and his colleagues on the island of Kos in Greece. That was more than 2500 years ago. Despite being a follower of Asclepius, the god of medicine, Hippocrates was the first to dismiss the idea that illness was caused or cured by superstitions and gods. He was the person that made medicine an art based on close observation, rational investigation with an emphasis on the concept 'First Do No Harm.'

As always in history, myths and their significance come and go on a pendulum. Sometimes they're buried, other times entangled with history, but we must get back to the narrative in difficult times, to help humanity face existential questions. If myths have been ignored for too long, people simply get lost and suffer from anomie. They are uprooted and suffer a breakdown of moral values.

Foundation myths are not dependent on culture or history; they transcend humanity. Myths are universal and timeless. During the Western Middle Ages, Christianity and its excess blurred medical history with a lot of unknown. They neglected the previous scientific knowledge including that embedded in the oath. Thereafter, during the Renaissance, intellectuals and artists discovered ancient Greek culture and opened their minds to rationality beyond religion, which began at the time of the antique Golden Age, on the 5th century BC. However, little is known about the oath's interpretation and use during the Renaissance. Closer to our time, due to the lack of following the oath, the world experienced severe atrocities. In the beginning of the twentieth century, the CDC led the Tuskegee Syphilis Study, and universities led human radiation experiments in the United States. In Europe, Nazi medical experiments were conducted without anyone stopping them, leading to the torture and death of millions of people.

Following the Second World War, people were shocked and needed to make sense of it all. How did this happen? How could scientists have been infected by evil banality? The Hippocratic oath and its myth came back to the rescue, not only as a way to understand what happened but also to prevent such abominations from ever happening again. The Declaration of Geneva, strongly inspired by the oath, was written and accepted worldwide as a code of conduct for all medical practitioners. It was first published in 1948.

I believe that today is the time for the oath's revival once more. The medical profession has become a cold science at risk of the banality of evil. Anomie must be fought against. We must preserve what makes us human and what makes us care. You see Melo, without caring for one another, human beings are doomed to fail. Hippocrates knew this. It's why the irrevocable rule was and always will be 'First Do No Harm.' The primordial myths are universal and timeless. They are here to rescue us again and again. We are only ever at the beginning, and the future belongs to those who remember how we began."

Melo listened so intently that she almost forgot the doctor was speaking in an altered voice.

"I've never worked in medicine before."

"I'm not asking you to work in medicine, I'm asking you to listen to my stories about the medical field and write with me."

"Ok."

"So then, we have a deal?"

"I think we do."

There was stillness between the two for a long moment. Melo finally examined what she could see in detail: a long, blood-red dress underneath a black hoody with the zip partly opened, bare legs and dark red socks above black Underground creepers in a London post-punk style. The doctor's hands drew Melo's attention. Her slender fingers were gracefully spread over the wood of the table, each of them decked with a silver ring: two in the shape of snakes, one Indian chief, one grim reaper, and one ring holding a skull and the face of a woman together in a kiss. An unusual doctor indeed.

Dr. Elpis reached her hand of rings into a black leather bag at her waist to retrieve a single scroll. She unrolled it. Melo recognised the paper from some of her father's illustrated encyclopaedias. It looked like an ancient illustration with gilded borders. It appeared as if it had been touched by every time period. Just as Melo was getting into it, the doctor scrolled it back up, and gently grabbed her hand and placed the scroll within it.

"This is the Hippocratic oath, Melo. For the next three months, it is yours and only yours. Keep good care of it and read it often. We will return to it every time we speak."

And as the doctor stood to leave the table at The Mirage, Melo exclaimed, almost involuntarily, "Wait, Doctor Elpis!"

The doctor's hood turned towards her.

"Will I ever hear your real voice?"

And at that moment, Dr. Elpis pulled the mic away from her face and spoke with the softest voice Melo had ever heard.

"We will make it just as you like Melo. I'll see you soon."

And then, she left.

Saturday one

Melo entered the library. The room was illuminated by the French windows facing the garden. Three sun rays penetrated the room in a nearly horizontal direction. Her father's desk on the opposite side of the window was in the semi-dark. The desk was filled with various books and papers with notes scribbled all over them. The open pink and ivory marble chimney was silent on the warm summer day. Above the chimney hung three Japanese masks, two *Hakushiko Noh,* and in the centre, a *Rojo Noh* mask representing a beautiful, aged poetess. The two *Hakushiko* masks were identical and bore the same soft smile, symbolising the world at peace.

Melo's father bought them in 1975 in New York following the death of his own father, John. Melo's grandfather was a prisoner of war in the Nagasaki Shipyard. He was one of the British soldiers captured at the battle of Singapore in 1942. The man had survived nearly four years of starvation, daily humiliation, recurrent tropical ulcers and dysentery. When he got back to the UK, he stayed in the Middlesex Hospital for six months. He got better though, and fell in love with Betty, one of the nurses. Betty was very special, she had a striking French accent and voluminous, curly, red hair. She was the best to dress his tropical ulcer, so much so that John used to joke that she cured him from it. Love devised the rest of their story.

Melo's father was born the following year. However, John kept physical sequelae of his past life. He sadly developed chronic anaemia, gastric ulcers and high blood pressure. He never spoke a word about his experiences in the Nagasaki Shipyard, but only said again and again, "I have already died." Sadly, a major stroke defeated him at the tender age of fifty.

To make sense of it all, Melo's father contacted an association of Prisoners of War and developed an interest for Japanese culture alongside his Greek linguistic studies. He wanted to understand his father. One day in New York, historical irony brought him to an antique shop run by the son of a Japanese-American locked down at the Ellis Island internment camp set up by Roosevelt following the Pearl Harbor attack. The two sons talked to each other and confabulated. They both shared their lack of grasp on what happened to their respective fathers. Respect and common ground appeared; sympathy happened. Melo's father eagerly bought the three *Eno* masks to ever remember this encounter.

That day, Melo's father sat silently, busy with his pipe smoking preparation on the velvet sofa. Melo crossed the room, stepping with catlike stealth over the indigo and ivory Persian rug that depicted a beautifully woven tree of life. She sat next to her father and unrolled the oath that Dr. Elpis had given her. She laid it flat on the wooden coffee table in front of them, carefully placing a small, smooth black stone on each of the four corners. Melo's father leaned over the oath and read it.

"This is a translation."

"It's not the original?"

"No, the original was written on clay tablets at the time of the Golden Age, in the 5th century BC. Copies written on papyrus burned in the Alexandria Library. However, the oath survived and got translated in Latin, Persian, Arabic and then in English and other modern languages all over the world. What you have got today is the first English translation by Francis Adam in 1849."

"She said that the oath had been forgotten several times in history, but she did not tell me about the original burning."

"What did she want from you?"

"She wants me to write about her experiences, I think, as a doctor. She kept talking about the world being in danger, about anomie affecting youth and that the oath was the answer. It was strange, she was in a hood, she had a voice changer. But I'm not sure why,

I just trusted her."

"So where do you go from here?"

"She's asked me to meet her every Saturday morning at The Mirage. She said every week she will tell new stories. I will listen and then write."

"What have I always told you?"

"That I would change the world."

"Yes, but what have I always told you about the myths?"

"As much as we rewrite the story, the story will always be the same."

"Correct. The principles which we found and create stories on are only ever different iterations of our origin stories. This is why I taught you through them as a child."

Melo remembered these teachings well. She let them guide her in every decision she ever made. She was home-schooled from the age of eight, pulled from primary school because she was not socialising properly. Her parents consulted the school psychologist who wrongly diagnosed autism. Her father and mother did not think twice: they pulled her out of the system at once. Her father was not impressed by the teaching of the time in any case, and simply disliked the intervention of psychologists at school. He decided to educate his daughter at home, away from these know-it-all headshrinkers as he used to call them. Her mother agreed with him from the start. The woman trusted her husband and relied on him for Melo's education. He believed he could do better than the teachers anyway. He knew Melo was special.

Melo wouldn't learn that she had Asperger's until she went to university at Durham to study social anthropology. There, she took the teachings of her father and her gifts as a writer to expand her mind. She started the blog when she was twenty-one. She didn't want to change anything or anyone, she began because she loved writing. It was her way of expressing herself.

"First Do No Harm."

"What about it?" Her dad inquired.

"The doctor kept repeating it."

"As someone that has read and heard of the oath from a linguistic perspective, 'do no harm' is the core value alongside confidentiality, respect, and other existential issues."

Melo's father watched as his child stared into the scroll as if it represented the entire universe. Melo's immediate interest and passion for the project were obvious to him. The man knew his child well. She was still fragile in social contexts, she was shy, yet on her own terms, was able to think and write beautifully. Melo had talent which needed the right impetus, and the doctor's project seemed appropriate.

"Melo."

"Yes."

"It does not require many words to speak the truth."

"Who said that?"

"Chief Joseph from the Nez Perce Tribe from the Pacific Northwest. Melo, it is the principle of the myths to be timeless in simplicity. As humans evolve and create more technology—and make this cacophony of ideas—the truth will never change but will just get buried in difficult times. It is us that must dig it out."

Melo thought about her own truths she held dear, like her love for her father, and how she found herself to be a writer. She thought about her mother too, and how she had such a hard time accepting the truth of her initial diagnosis of autism. She remembered watching her mother speak to people in their community about her, "I have heard it could be genetic, but no one in my family has ever had such an issue," or "it is not her fault she is an aspie, a kind of bright autist, you know." Melo knew her mother's ignorance well, she sympathised with her inability to understand and her need to find a reason or excuse for why she was different. Besides, her mother came to terms with it in time. Time is a healer.

Melo gently pushed the four black stones off the oath and rolled it back up. She stood from the red velvet sofa and said goodnight to her father.

▲

Melo took the underground from Richmond to Oxford Circus for a second time. She studied all week. She took her conversation with her father and read the oath repeatedly, preparing for the next meeting with Elpis.

Melo walked up the escalator and eagerly crossed the circus in a diagonal. She was heading for The Mirage once again. London on Saturday morning was unusually calm and empty. She was shocked once again how the atmosphere could change so extremely based on the day of the week. It was eerie to be walking almost all alone in the epicentre of the metropolis.

She walked down Noel and then Poland Street, crossed Berwicks Lane and readied herself to enter the restaurant at exactly 6:57 am. She opened the door and crossed the dark room through the narrow space of the bar underneath the stone ceilings, following the path that the Mia look-alike had taken her along the week before.

"Good morning, Melo. The doctor is waiting for you. What would you like to drink?"

The voice of the waitress came from behind the bar as Melo turned to meet her eyes. She felt her cheeks blush, hunched over to let her curls cover her cheeks and walked on as if she hadn't heard the voice of the waitress at all.

She reached the doctor's table and sat down immediately. Behind her, the waitress didn't think anything of it and just went on with the preparation of the matcha tea.

Doctor Elpis was sitting, back straight with her ring-filled hands intertwined at the table. It was like the doctor had not left at all. With the same soft and gentle voice, she said, "Good morning, Melo. Good timing. How are you today? Have you read the oath?"

"I have, Doctor. I read it many times. I shared it with my father, who is a linguist by profession. You will be happy to know that he agreed with your choice of translation, and more importantly, with our project."

The Mia Wallace look-alike brought the matcha tea.

Melo looked sincerely into the waitress's eyes and said thank you with a nod of her head.

Doctor Elpis pulled a piece of paper from her black leather bag once again and placed it on the table between the two of them. This paper was not an old-fashioned scroll, but a piece of stationary paper. The top of the document was entitled 'Elpis and Melo Schedule.'

Melo saw the oath broken down into twelve different parts, each associated with the date of a meeting. The first meeting on the page was unrelated to any full part of the oath, it only said 'Meeting One, Do No Harm.'

"This is my plan for us. Each meeting, a story or a series of stories will coincide with a part of this oath. Today is the beginning. 'I swear by Apollo the physician, and Asclepius, and Health, and All-heal, and all the gods and goddesses, that, according to my ability and judgment, I will keep this oath and this stipulation.' Are you ready?"

"Yes, I think so."

Melo pulled her Moleskine notebook and pen from her backpack and titled the page 'Story Number One'.

And the doctor began.

"I was not born to be a doctor and faith had nothing to do with my destiny. However, very early on, I found the vocation and discovered the universal wisdom attached to my profession. There were three events which impacted my destiny. The first was when I was a child of seven.

One morning, I was running in the fields on my own. My brothers and sisters were still sleeping. I was running in a sweetcorn field, in the northeast of my village in Brittany, France called Ploumilliau. I was heading to the hedgerows where in my imaginary world, I was an Indian and surveying the land with my comrades. I was very skilled at climbing the branches of trees and considered myself a courageous warrior. People called me '*yeux perçants*', piercing eyes, because I was considered such a good observer.

However, to be considered an observer did not satisfy me, I wished to be more than that. Sometimes in this world I would escape to, I would bring my siblings with me. My brother Simon would play the chief of the village, and I would play the shaman, the healer. I dreamt of being by his side and caring for the chief. That was my sole ambition.

But that day, in my imaginary world, I was on my own. When I reached the other side of the sweetcorn field, I ducked underneath the electric barrier, and took the secret passage along the hedge-row. I'd imagine the solemn scene of a peace pipe ceremony around me, watching the old shaman and the chiefs speak about my rite of passage as I listened and watched in admiration of what I hoped to become. As I sat and imagined the conversation, a peculiar noise alerted me. Something was rustling on the side of an alder's trunk. I stood and approached the tree silently, with the utmost care. As I walked to the back side of the tree, I saw a bird lying down on its side with a bloody wing flapping. I got closer. It appeared that only one of the wings had been injured. The bird moved spasmodically for a few seconds and then stopped. It was September and the sweetcorn was high and ready for harvesting. The bird, like others, should have been ready for the long flight back to the coastline of Morocco and Senegal, and on to Africa. I knew that well, for my mother had told me so. The bird and I were surrounded by billowing skirts of blackthorns, dog roses, and bramble filled with blackberries. I felt a part of the life sources that surrounded me that day, and I felt a duty of care. I gazed into the injured bird's eyes as the bird looked into mine. Maybe it had been hurt by a heedless young buzzard not skilled enough to catch its prey properly.

I inspected the bird. Even now, I remember the black and white striped patch on the neck. I suspected it to be a *tourterelle des bois*, or turtle dove because it was smaller than the pigeons living in my courtyard and larger than the blackbirds.

I pulled out my multi-coloured, twenty-nine centimetre long handkerchief and wrapped the bird, careful not to hurt the injured wing. I picked up the animal and held it against my well-fed stomach, just above the belly button, underneath my coat to keep it warm and safe. I trailed back home like a scavenger and kept the bird steady and close to my body.

It was the morning still, and on that particular day, there was no school. My brothers and sisters were still asleep when I got home, but the table was already set for breakfast. There were blue and yellow bowls on the chequered, red and white cotton tablecloth, with spoons to the right and red napkins on the left. In the centre of the table was a large lump of butter alongside the chocolate powder container, and a pot of homemade blackberry jam. A freshly baked three-pound loaf of bread sat to the side of the butter, and the scent of coffee and cooked apples filled the air.

My mother was in the kitchen, busy plucking the still warm beheaded chicken. There was a large, red enamel basin at her side, containing fresh milk I'd collected from the neighbourhood farm the night before. I did not mind my mother plucking; however, I couldn't wait to watch her remove the clotted cream from the milk. I liked to see how the cream broke at the surface into various geometric shapes, and sometimes I could catch a rainbow from the light entering through the interstice between the milk and the creamy surface.

As I tiptoed closer to the table, my mother turned to find me.

'Elpis, what have you gotten up to? Your brothers and sisters are still sleeping.'

I slowly unveiled my jacket to reveal the colourfully wrapped bird. My mother did not respond with words but went to get a box for me. When she returned, I softly pulled the bird from my coat, and unwrapped it gently from the multi-coloured handkerchief. I cautiously placed the bird in the box. It barely moved. I worried this would soon be the end, but when I placed a small plate of water next to the bird, it reached its beak out to take a sip. I knew there was hope. I cleaned the bird's wing, feather by feather until the bleeding stopped. But it was weak. I knew—even though I was young—that an injured animal unable to stand and unwilling to escape would most likely die.

And the day went on. I played with my sisters and brothers, and from time to time, we all went to see the bird. I was in charge, though.

Twilight settled in around the little home by the sweetcorn field when I went to check again and sadly found my turtle dove inanimate and dead."

A silence washed through the back of The Mirage between the two women.

Realising that the story was over, Melo proclaimed,

"Is that it?"

"Yes."

"But what happened to the bird?"

"The bird died later that day."

"So sad. Did that not change your perspective on helping?"

"Caring, Melo, is not about saving lives. It's about giving hope. It's about making the moments, especially if they are the last, as comfortable as they can be. That bird died wrapped in warmth with water by its side. And that was all I could do."

Melo let this sit. She understood that the stories the doctor would tell were up to her to find the moral principle within. The doctor carried on, without a moment's hesitation.

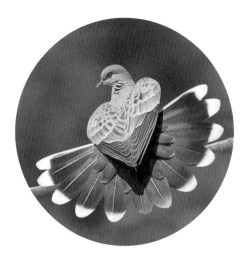

"At the age of nine, I was running through the corridors of my home with my sister. As we ran, my sister began twirling her jacket in the air in circular motions pretending she was a gymnast doing a ribbon dance routine. On her jacket was a string of metal buttons, and as she spun, one of them met my eye. My eyelid was bruised, and turned purple very quickly, but I went on as if nothing happened. A few days later, I woke in the middle of the night with a horrible headache. I tried to open my eyes but could not. I went to my mother's room and stood at the edge of the bed, I put my hand in front of my right eye and declared, "Maman, look, I cannot see any more with this eye." I was instantly brought back to bed, given some water, and told to go back to sleep until the morning.

The next day, I was taken to an eye specialist, an ophthalmologist consultant in town. We arrived and waited with the other patients before being welcomed into the consulting room. In the room were a large desk and machinery. I was examined in silence with a square, black apparatus called a slit lamp. The ophthalmologist did a comprehensive examination, checking my eye pressure. He then revealed to my mother and I that I was suffering with a hyphema, a pooling of blood inside the space between the cornea and the iris. If left untreated, I could have permanent loss of vision. He handed me an eyepatch and sent us to the hospital on the spot. We were told I had to lie down at all times with my head elevated at least forty degrees, or I could lose my eyesight forever.

As I walked in, holding my mother's hand, I looked out into the hospital room with my one eye and took in my surroundings. I saw the white walls, and sterile floor below the big windows. The white bed felt like a throne. And the room smelt unlike anything I'd ever come across before: like all the dirt in the world was absorbed and destroyed in that large, bright space. Now, I'd say it was like chloroform or ether and I loved it! Nurses would come and check on me like my mother would. I was not concerned about having a scar because if I had one then I'd have something to remember the hospital by.

Each day, I was brought on a stretcher to have my eye pressure checked by the doctor. The daily visit to the darkroom was exquisite. As soon as I entered the examination room, the doctor would already be in position in front of the slit lamp. He would be wearing a long, white coat and tie, and his hands, his hands were the complete opposite of everything I knew. There were no dirty cuticles, shaved down skin, cuts or bruises. His hands were clean. They were perfectly clean. I could have sworn they were shining. They were very agile too. I would watch his hands pull the apparatus down and see how delicately and skilled they'd move. I wished to use my hands like that. And as a little girl, I trusted this doctor fully. There was no fear, only a desire to stay.

The treatment was a success. After ten days, the pressure in my eye normalised, all the blood trapped between the cornea and the iris dissipated as predicted. The patch was removed, and I could see again."

Melo looked up at the doctor, realising the story was over.

"Did you ever go to a hospital again?"

"I wouldn't end up back in hospital until I myself trained to be a doctor. Are you ready for the next story, Melo?

Melo nodded and went back to taking notes.

"At the age of twenty, I was in my foundation year training to be a doctor in Paris. It was at this time that the AIDS epidemic started. I entered medical school in 1983. I was doing ward rounds with my classmates, the professor and fellow doctors. We would walk up and down through the ward, checking on patients and learning by watching the doctor's work. We would listen to them discuss the cases of each patient and develop our medical language and knowledge. Sometimes, we'd be put on the spot and asked to assist doctors with certain patients.

I was called once to help a patient and do blood work. I already considered this routine and went at once. I walked through the hall, looking for Room 12 which held a patient named Jacques Du Mougin. I was rushing through when I saw him for the first time. And I will never forget that sight. A Hippocratic face with a leaden complexion and sunken eyes. The man behind the face was lying down in the hospital bed and was about to die. Jacques was sat on the bed, his eyes gauging from his head, looking up at the wall, looking at nothing. He was emaciated, only bones, barely skin.

I was paralysed for a moment, putting together the shocking site, the sadness of the situation and my duties. I then went forward as usual.

I stepped into the room and said, 'Hello Jacques, my name is Elpis. I am going to take care of your blood test today. How are you doing?'

He could barely speak full sentences. He tried to smile with his dry, white lips and tongue but I knew it took too much from him to bring his lips to curl and bare his teeth. But he cooperated with ease. I assured him he would feel no pain, and I did not ask him anything other than what I needed to know to do my job.

Jacques was about to die from AIDS, a new disease that nobody had a cure for. Panacea was not with us. But worse happened. Around me, opinions and judgements related by the media were spreading as fast as the epidemic. Stigmatisation aggravated the predicaments of those affected by AIDS.

When high-profile people started contracting the disease, the media began representing it as if it was the consequence of people seeking out sexual liberation and in doing so prompted the weakening of the idea of private life, intimacy and medical secrecy.

The fate of Freddy Mercury springs to mind. He had AIDS and kept the diagnosis away from the media till the end. His condition was not revealed to the media by the doctors, secrecy was respected. He was fully aware of his end approaching and the doctors stayed at his bedside, respecting his privacy. Only two days before his death, Freddy committed an act of courage which will live on in history.

The beloved rock singer from Queen, the creator of the iconic *Bohemian Rhapsody*, revealed to the public his incurable condition only a few hours before dying. His doctors were aware of the prognosis; they were helping the star with palliative care as the singer made a courageous move. Freddy knew his death was approaching, yet he did not ask to die. Rather, he decided to address his fans and the general public with the hope that his sacrifice may help others in the future. He told them:

'I wish to confirm that I have been tested HIV positive and have AIDS … the time has come now for my friends and fans around the world to know the truth and I hope that everyone will join with me, my doctors and all those worldwide in the fight against this terrible disease.'

His address was an act of courage on the brink of death, which came a few hours later, in one moment, a final point, one single instant in time, with a 'before' and an 'after'.

At the time of Freddy Mercury's death, we still had a limited understanding of the science behind AIDS, but that did not change the doctors' sense of duty to care.

Melo, Jacques Du Mougin was like Freddy Mercury. The man was in my mind a patient like everyone else, a human being who was suffering and who needed to be cared for. I did not need to know how he got there. I did not need the science to care for him and respect his dignity. In my profession, we use judgment only to assess, diagnose and treat. There is no room for prejudice. Judgment is limited to observation and care. Observation and care."

A strange silence gently settled. Melo waited to see if the doctor had another for her that day. But she remained silent.

"Thank you for today, Melo. I look forward to seeing you next Saturday when we move onto the next part of the oath."

And as one woman stood to leave, the other soon followed. The first meeting had come to an end.

▲

Melo was ready to leave. The young woman opened her bedroom window and watched as a plane crossed the cloudless, blue sky leaving a straight white line behind it. Birds whistled a continuous melody, bridged at random by beeps and clicks. Melo listened.

A nascent wind agitated the tree leaves lit and engorged with sunshine. The woman, still listening, took a big breath of fresh air and went back to her backpack. She carefully wrapped up the Hippocratic oath back in the sky-blue tissue paper that she fastened the night before and placed it inside her backpack. She grabbed one of her jumpers and placed it around the oath for extra protection, and loosely closed the top of the backpack. She placed her notebook and pen box in the back pocket. She locked her phone and tucked it into the front pocket. Melo was ready to go. Downstairs, her mother and father were quietly sitting at the breakfast table reading the weekend newspapers.

Melo went to kiss her parents on the cheek goodbye.

"Have a good day," her mother said.

"That's my girl. Don't work too hard, promise," the father said, gazing above the frame of his glasses at her leaving the room.

"You know I will! Goodbye!"

Melo left through the front door. She crossed the garden, opened the gate and walked down Richmond Avenue. The streets were quiet on that Saturday morning. Only two joggers passed by, running and pacing themselves to their music.

For the third meeting with the doctor, Melo felt in control. She had spent the week researching the oath, breaking it down line by line and reading through the history. She started with the beginning.

"I swear by Apollo the physician, and Asclepius and Hygeia and Panacea"

She knew Apollo since she was a kid as the beautiful multipower god at the origin of everything, but the other three she'd not heard of. She knew Hygeia, or rather the name. Hygeia was the goddess of cleanliness, and her name was the root for the word hygiene. Panacea was a goddess whose name meant 'remedy for everything'. Elpis referred to it last week when she said doctors did not have the panacea at the beginning of the AIDS epidemic. Hygeia and Panacea were sisters and the daughters of Asclepius.

Melo had never heard of Asclepius. She discovered that he was the god of medicine, not Hippocrates. Like Hercules, he was a demigod born from Apollo and a mortal called Coronis. Asclepius was taken away from his mother at birth because of her infidelity. He was raised by Chiron, the wisest and fairest centaur who taught him the secrets together with his guardians, the snakes.

Five days ago, her father found an illustrated book in the library. He remembered. He bought it at the Waterstones bookshop in Bloomsbury a few days after his visit of the Vatican Museums in Rome. This was in 2008, he recalled. His eyes were caught by the cover page of the book set up on the new table dedicated for second-hand books at Waterstones. A statue of Asclepius holding his wooden staff with an entwined snake tight to his body was pictured. The style resembled one of the statues he admired at the Vatican Museums. It was the same facture, the same era, or the same artist. The title of the book was *Asclepius: The God of Medicine* and was written by Dr. Gerald D Hart, a Canadian doctor.

Dr. Hart was not only a passionate doctor but also an expert numismatist. As a result, the book was illustrated with many photos of coins, votives, altars and other antique relics from various European areas where Asclepius was venerated.

In the introduction, Dr. Hart mentioned that the very name of the god of medicine had two etymologies: 'heal gently' and 'deferring the dryness that comes from death,' and that both meanings were fundamental to his profession's very roots and foundation myth.

Her father read that according to the myth, the snakes were the guardians of the young Asclepius. They taught him the secrets of the medicinal properties of plants. He said to Melo that in antiquity, snakes were often domesticated but also venerated as the symbol of life, transcendence and renewal. The snake was a quasi-omnipresent figure in the ancient time. Many Greek gods were represented in association with snakes, from Medusa, Athena, Apollo, Hygeia and Asclepius of course. Hermes' caduceus, a rod with two snakes entwined, has often been mistaken as the symbol of medicine, which of course, it is not.

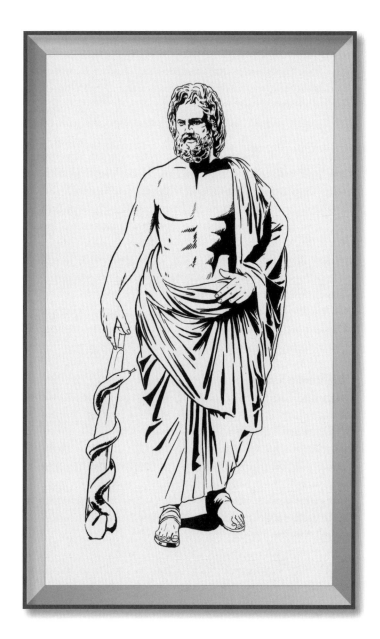

Furthermore, according to the book, snakes were part of the scene in temples dedicated to Asclepius and played a role in rituals and cures. Incubation was known as the most frequent healing ritual practiced in these ancient times. It consisted of a night in the temple with priests, snakes and dogs wandering around. The temple was immaculate and clean, the priests wore a fine, white net in their hair and an immaculate himation. Cleanliness was paramount, so much so that plagues never entered the edifices. Patients were cleaned thoroughly with a bath the night before. The temples were spectacular, filled with huge statues of Asclepius, and tablets or votives with numerous patient testimonials lined on the wall as decoration. Music was played to heal the mind. This setup was meant to induce dreams involving Asclepius and often people were cured from their illness as a result.

Melo examined at length an illustration of a bas-relief of a patient receiving treatment to his shoulder at the temple. It was a vis-à-vis depicting two separate events or two interpretations of what happened. At the forefront, a doctor was treating the shoulder of a standing patient. In the background, the same patient was lying down asleep with a snake biting his right shoulder, while a priest was praying or incanting at his bedside.

Was the doctor Asclepius? In that case, the patient dreamt of Asclepius and believed that he was cured as a result. Or was the doctor a physician, like Hippocrates, who came to the temple to treat the man following the ritual of incubation?

Asclepius was the god of medicine, not Hippocrates. Hippocrates has never been a god or a mythical entity, that is a proven historical truth. He, nevertheless, collaborated with the priests in the temple.

Hippocrates lived during the Golden Age of Athens in the 5th century BC. This was a period of peace, harmony, stability and prosperity which brought the first ever democracy on Earth. As Elpis mentioned previously, he was the physician who developed medical care based on science and observation alongside rituals based on tradition. That was now clear in Melo's mind.

To reckon him who taught me this Art equally
dear to me as my parents, to share my substance
with him, and relieve his necessities if required;
to look upon his offspring in the same footing as my
own brothers, and to teach them this Art, if they
shall wish to learn it, without fee or stipulation;
and that by precept, lecture, and every other mode
of instruction, I will impart a knowledge of the
Art to my own sons, and those of my teachers,
and to disciples bound by a stipulation and oath
according to the law of medicine, but to none others

HIPPOCRATES

Saturday Two

Melo was thinking of the connections between Dr. Elpis, Hippocrates, Asclepius and his snake when she emerged from the Oxford Circus underground station. A plane was darting above her through the blue sky as she walked down Carnaby Street. One man on the other side of the street walked along the sidewalk with one AirPod in, talking to the emptiness inside his head.

6:57 am. Melo walked faster. She could *not* be late.

Soho was sleeping after another crazy night of debauchery, she thought. Melo passed Greek Street and the Crowbar: a small dark pub where rock and metal was played from a jukebox. She'd never had a night out there, but she'd like to. Her friends from the band told her about it. 6.59 am, Melo opened the door of The Mirage frantically, about to set off towards the meeting place in the back when the Mia look-alike caught her eyes.

"Good morning, Melo."

Melo smiled at the sight of her unfamiliar new friend. She wished to know her, but never felt comfortable being the one to start a conversation. Being home-schooled isolated her from most of the young kids of her age. It wasn't until university that she would be surrounded by people. Her mates know she has Asperger's but actually did not take any notice of it. In any case, this never felt like a real issue to Melo. It was who she was, who she always was. But sometimes, when she would tell her peers, she'd watch them withdraw, unsure of how to move forward. She saw that they believed her to be different from them, and never made the effort to understand her. Throughout school she'd had acquaintances, but Melo never had a true friend, really. The members of her band were, just like her, all emerged in their occupations and music.

She walked on as a blush beautifully lit her face. Her shoulders fell forward and she murmured, "Hi" to the waitress.

She continued to the back of The Mirage and found Doctor Elpis sat before her cappuccino. Melo sat promptly, let out a sigh, and found the doctor with her eyes.

"Dearest Melo, it's nice to see you again. I told the waitress to get you a matcha, is that alright?"

"Yes. Thank you. I spent the week reading and speaking with my father about Asclepius. Do you know what his name translates to?"

"Heal gently."

"It has a second meaning as well, did you know that?"

"No. What is it?"

"Deferring the dryness that comes from death."

"Where did you get that?"

"My father. He has a book, written by a doctor, called *Asclepius: the God of Medicine*."

"Melo, it always fascinated me how the meaning of language changes with time. The two phrases mean the same thing, essentially. When one is close to death, the skin and muscles begin to dry up. But life on Earth is the opposite of dryness; we are 90% water. My profession has to do with preventing and delaying that process of dryness. To bring some moisture back is being kind, it is delaying and reducing the suffering. At some point in our life, we all confront the risk of death, Melo. But death should be one moment, not a continuous battle.

I have confronted death many times in my life. Not only with my loved ones, some artists I used to love, but also my patients.

My brother Vivian died before my mother. He was only thirteen and I was seven. He simply had tonsillitis, the doctor had given him an antibiotic to make it go away. However, in a few hours, my brother developed a major allergy to the supposed cure. After taking his first dose, my mother sent him to bed to rest. Later, she asked me to check on him and see if he wanted dinner. When I went to his room, he woke up and began to make a sound from his throat. He was heaving and groaning, but I did not realise anything was wrong. I was only seven. I left and went to my room to collect my dolly, and the last thing I heard was my brother rushing and falling down the stairs to the kitchen. I ran down to follow, and saw my mother holding him, trying to open his mouth. She shouted at me to go get my stepfather for help. He came, picked up my brother, and the three of them left for the hospital. But it was too late when they arrived. My brother had passed. He was allergic to various things not identified at that time. That antibiotic put him into an anaphylactic shock. He had symptoms previously of less serious allergic reactions like urticaria, nettle rash, and oedema. But this one was fatal. Back then, medical care was not part of family life like it is now. We did not have the resources or even the knowledge. What my brother needed was an adrenaline pen, and a doctor now would have known to test for allergies.

I don't speak of that experience much, but it has affected how I am as a doctor. I have spent much of my career terrified of mis-prescribing medication.

Today, I want to speak on what the oath teaches us on how to go through painful life events while caring for each other guided by the oath, not only doctor to patient, but doctor to doctor.

I am conscious that I live my life with the privilege of not having to think of the inescapable until another day, and another time, and another incident. My work, habits, family, relationships, duties, regulations, bills, etc, carry on, one after another.

However, recently, I have had to face a succession of dramas. The sequence started with a patient who collapsed in my practice with a brain haemorrhage.

I resuscitated him so that he survived that near-death experience. I was shaky for several weeks following the event. Life is indeed so fragile, I thought. But I carried on, as always, with days following one another, until I was once again confronted with the possibility of an imminent death. Another patient came in and told me about a pain across his chest that had happened a few days before while snorkelling in the Maldives among guitarfish, whiprays, and butterfly fish. He described the exact pain of a heart attack I had read about in my medical textbooks and that I have seen on several occasions. I ran the routine tests, but to my surprise, all came back normal. However, I knew something was wrong. My instinct and my skills were at stake. I said to the man that all his tests were normal, but that he needed to see a cardiologist consultant immediately. Later, he was diagnosed with a massive myocardial infarction, a heart attack. The man had a partial blockage which made his arteries go into spasm; however, this makes the artery at risk of going into a full blockage. If this happens, the person can die within minutes. I told him not to go home despite the normal results, and in doing so, I saved his life. The artery got fully blocked at the time he was with the cardiologist who was able to treat him on the spot.

For the following weeks, I was shaken once again. I became acutely aware that I must go through these dangerous moments as a doctor, and then move on. And I did, until one day something happened to me. The day I went to have my routine mammogram.

I must admit that I do not like the test, in which my small breasts are squeezed into a machine. The idea of it is unpleasant, a bit scary and a little painful. But I went. I had to.

The dreaded medical investigation went well. The operator was kind and experienced in the matter. She skilfully manipulated both the human breast and the machine and things went on smoothly. After just ten minutes, I was free to go back to normal life. Later that day, the operator called my office.

'Hello, Dr. Elpis, there is a problem with your mammogram, you need to come back and have an ultrasound.'

A bit taken aback, I replied, 'Ok, when would you like me to come?'

'We can actually see you tomorrow morning, at 8 am.'

'Oh thanks, that'll do.'

After putting the phone down, I thought, *I know, I have got dense breasts, that's why,* and then did not think any more about it and got back to work.

Next morning, 8 am.

'Good morning. Thank you for seeing me so early.'

As instructed, I, the patient, took off my clothes from the waist up and laid down on the medical couch. My colleague, the radiologist, then entered the room.

'Good morning, Dr. Elpis. Let's see what the problem is.' The doctor sat down in front of a big screen, holding the sonar in her right hand. Some gel was then applied around the probe and moved gently on and around my breast. Carefully, she checked the left and then the right, probing at different angles, again and again. What was she doing? Taking some measurements? Of what? Why? This carried on and on; I was getting nervous when the silence was broken.

'Elpis, there is a lump, I need to take a biopsy. I can do that now.'

'What? What did you say, a lump? Are you sure? This cannot be. I'm sorry, this just cannot be.'

'Yes, Dr. Elpis, there is a lump, the mammogram is showing it too. It may be nothing to worry about, but we need to do a biopsy.'

'No, I cannot, I have to go, patients are waiting for me.'

I stood up and grabbed my clothes. The nurse held my arm and said, 'This can be done in a few minutes, it won't hurt.'

'No, I am sorry, this is just impossible, I have to go.' I dressed quickly without saying a word. Then, I murmured, 'I have to go to my patients now.'

The nurse took my hand sympathetically, gazed intensely at me and said, 'Doctor, promise me you'll call this afternoon to fix another time, promise me please.'

'Okay, I will,' I replied, hesitantly.

I escaped, rushing outside of the damn breast clinic and, in a few minutes, I was in my office building on the other side of Harley Street. Alice, the receptionist, saw me entering the building. At first sight, she understood something had happened. I looked at her as tears began welling in my eyes.

I froze, looked at her, and no noise came out of my mouth. I tried to say, 'They want to biopsy my breast' but only my lips moved. I then walked further towards her, took the friendly hand and said,

'They want to biopsy my breast, I've got cancer.' Then, I walked away, holding my tears back with determination, and entered my office and closed the door behind me.

While at my desk, I did not cry. There was no time for it. No, I got back to my senses quickly and got on with my work. I saw patients one after another, like any other day. Later, Alice found an opportunity to speak to me.

'It is a test, that does not mean you have cancer. I know many friends who've had biopsies, do not worry.'

I thanked her for her words and sympathy and then called my colleague to arrange a time for the bloody biopsy. And the next day, I went. I walked back into the examination room and removed my clothes again from the waist up and lay down on the couch on my right side as instructed. My radiologist colleague stood in front of a big screen with the probe in his hand, as the nurse stood by with all necessary materials to perform the biopsy. I turned my head to face the wall as one, tiny painful punch hit my body, my small, lovely breast got punctured. They removed some tissue from the lump and took it away. A bandage was immediately applied. The biopsy was over. An appointment was then made for the following week with the breast surgeon, Mr. Machaon. I was free to go.

I hurried back to my office and back to being the doctor. The following week, I went back to speak to Mr. Machaon to hear what had been found.

'Elpis, it is cancer, we found it early, it is very small, and as you know we can treat it easily. You need a lumpectomy though. Can we do this next week?'

This time, I reacted objectively, factually. I gave all my trust to Mr. Machaon. It was trust at first sight. Of course, I knew the doctor already, but I could see and sense his confidence here, his skills and professional compassion kept me calm. I could be the patient, in all confidence. I could let go.

I asked, 'Can we delay the surgery to December? It will help me organise my work and Christmas time will be an opportunity to rest.'

'I cannot see any issue with that, let's do it.'

The arrangements were made. I called the insurance; I could sense the girl on the other side of the phone wanting to show empathy as I pronounced the word cancer. I could feel it. But I just did not want it. I just did not want empathy from a stranger. Just be professional.

Melo, my disease, my cancer was part of me, part of my intimate life. I did not wish to share it with strangers in any way, let alone over the phone. My cancer was mine, and I should be able to choose with whom I talked about it.

A few weeks later, I went back for the surgery. When I entered the building, a kind nurse from the Philippines welcomed me and showed me the room where I would rest and sleep following the procedure. They instructed me on the schedule for the day. I filled out the forms, they took my blood pressure, and then my surgeon entered the room. With sympathetic and reassuring words, Mr. Machaon examined me and drew an arrow on my right arm to indicate which side of my body was being attacked by the cancer, the side which needed surgical attention.

'We should be on time, Dr. Elpis, see you later.'

Within two minutes, he was gone, but he'd done his job. Once again, he had my trust. It was now the turn of the anaesthetist. He examined me, asked a few questions to the nurse, and said, 'See you soon, Dr. Elpis. All is well organised, we should be on time.'

I was confident as any patient in good hands would be and when the stretcher arrived, I was ready. Without being asked, I laid down. The man pushed the stretcher to the dedicated lift. The metallic grey door opened, the stretcher and I were gobbled up by it. The nurse stayed behind, and waved goodbye as the elevator doors closed. A few seconds later, the doors of the lift opened to a corridor. On the right-hand side was a large door which opened automatically into the operating theatre, where Mr. Machaon, the anaesthetist and a tall nurse were all busy setting up the scene. They helped to transfer my body from the stretcher to the operating table. The anaesthetist took my hand, and whispered a few gentle words …

Forty-five minutes later, I woke up, with him by my side. '*Les ganglions sont saints, ma chérie.*'

The cancer had not spread. Melo, I only remember those words, my contentment in hearing them, and the faint joy amongst the mist of anaesthetic. These six simple French words meant that my cancer had not spread to the lymph nodes. Together, these words meant that I was one of the lucky ones. The cancer had been picked up early enough not to need chemotherapy treatment. I would not lose my hair, I would not be incapacitated for six months, and I would be able to go back to work.

Back in my room, I slept in peace. In the morning, the nurse was by my side checking my blood pressure, temperature, and my breast's dressing. It was bleeding. She left me and came back a few moments later with Mr. Machaon.

'Elpis, I am sorry it is bleeding, I need to redo the dressing.'

'This does happen sometimes.'

The skilled surgeon then proceeded, with the help of the nurse, to fix the wrapping around my breast. He assured me he would be back tomorrow to check on me.

Mr. Machaon indeed came back and checked the bandage. It was immaculate. I was allowed to go back home. Home, sweet home. I could rest without any pain despite having to give up my preferred position to fall asleep. I actually slept like a log. However, three days later, I felt discomfort in my breast, which had become quite swollen. It did not bother me though. I decided that the swelling was quite normal and that I should be Ok. However, when I saw Mr. Machaon a few days later, the man shook his head in disappointment.

'I am so sorry, Dr. Elpis, you have a large hematoma. It needs to be drained.'

Out of sympathy, he held my arm, and moved his head ever so gently side to side and said, with a reassuring tone, 'We will sort this out.'

In an instant, he got to work around my breast. He opened the large incision and drained the excess fluid. I looked the other way. I could not gaze at the opening of my sick breast. I was alright though; I felt cared for.

After it was finished, I sat down and put my clothes back on. However, I could sense the doctor's weariness. He was more anxious than I was. I left the building reassured and positive. Things would be alright, I thought. I was convinced I would recover soon.

Thereafter, the hematoma did not come back and, as planned, I had radiotherapy and hormonal treatments. The radiotherapy sessions were all lined up to start a few weeks later. My breast and nipple reacted to the high energy X-ray beams. My skin became even more sore. I used the natural cream I had been given and followed the instructions exactly. However, it did not stop the pain, so I stopped wearing a bra, and then my elegant dresses, and I started to sleep on the other side of the bed. And time went on as it always has. My breast and nipple took weeks to improve but they did, and my life went on without physical pain. My cancer became part of my new life. I had a deeper empathy for those around me, I cherished my own life more.

Months passed, one after another, in my new self. I left London for a well-deserved rest in my home in Anjou, France. I was lucky, the Ronsard roses were blooming under a beautiful blue sky. It felt homely.

When I arrived, I was sitting comfortably on the velvet sofa. I was contemplating the garden through the window, looking at the lone, twisted, pale-pink eglantine. I was happy that it had survived the inadequacy of my planting in the garden. It was all alone, twisted but strong and blooming. And then he appeared to me. Hippocrates.

He was sitting comfortably in the blue armchair near the bay window. I looked at his quiet face with his porcelain skin. His white hair was beautifully curly. His nose was aquiline and his beard full and strikingly wavy. The father of medicine was wearing an immaculate and perfectly draped himation.

He stood from the armchair and smiled at me as he made his way to the stereo. He pressed the number 1, and *O Green World* from the band Gorillaz started playing through the room. He did not react, but quickly went back to sitting and picked up his lyre—to him it would be called a kithara—and sat in front of me. He began to play along to the song I knew so well. I felt the cells of my skin opening like butterflies. I could speak the truth.

I burst out.

'Hippocrates, during my treatment, I kept thinking of all my patients from the past. I could not stop remembering the ones who had to go through cancer treatment, their suffering, complaints and physical symptoms were coming back to my mind. I thought of the mother who told me about the plans she had for her children's future on the very day she died. All these memories came back to me while I was sick. Even when my breasts were in pain, my mind was still thinking of my previous patients. And now, beside these memories, I do not remember my own pain and suffering. Am I crazy?'

'You are not crazy, Dr. Elpis. You are a physician. Your work is embedded in your being.'

Hippocrates carried on playing his lyre. I relaxed, breathed deeply, rested and listened. The music was joined by a thrush and a Eurasian blackbird's melody from outside the room.

Hippocrates stood from the armchair, and said to me, "My dear Elpis, life is short. Let's go walking in the garden. Let us go outside and see the birds and the roses."

I put my old, blue-indigo pashmina around my shoulders and followed Hippocrates outside. We both looked up at the pine tree to catch a glimpse of the Eurasian blackbird. The thrush, who was so loud a few moments ago, was not to be seen. I gazed at my beloved Japanese maple tree and the twisted pink eglantine I planted with my own hands a few years before. We carried on walking, silently and peacefully, until my master held my arm and pointed with his other hand to the plum tree. I looked. A red squirrel was spiralling around the trunk. The small mammal was going up and down the tree over and over, and then stopped. It did not go up again but stayed still. Hippocrates, with his finger still pointed towards the tree, whispered to me, 'Dear Elpis, why has it stopped? Why has this tiny, wild animal with its ear tufts, bright, rusty red fur and bushy tail stopped its important business just now? Why?'

'He may have sensed our presence, Hippocrates, and is waiting to understand what our intentions may be.'

'My dear friend, the little, wild animal senses our presence indeed, but it is not worried about our intentions, not at all. The animal knows. Elpis, you have a mysterious and beautiful link with nature. Believe in it, connect with Earth and its inhabitants. Spread your kindness to humanity and nature, and let them both come back to you. Your colleagues have done their part according to the oath. I trust them. They have all shown scientific ability, talent, kindness, and wisdom, you can count on them all. And on your side, just connect your kindness to humanity and nature as you know to do it.

Hippocrates was right. It was time to return to reality.

Melo, Hippocrates is no more, and I will also die one day, but not too soon, I hope."

Silence settled around the two women at The Mirage. Dr. Elpis packed while uttering a few words. Something like "Melo, see you next week." The young woman acquiesced with a nod of her head letting her hair fall and cover her eyes. Melo did not know what to say. She was struck with a sudden all-encompassing vulnerability, and did not want to move yet as she watched the doctor go.

Mia approached.

"Hi, would you like another tea before leaving?"

"Not really. When are the regular customers coming?"

"Not before 10 am."

"Ok."

"Are you alright?"

"I am fine. Let's have tea, would you like one?"

"Yes, smashing. I'll bring the drinks."

Mia went. Melo stayed in the same position, deep in her thoughts. She still did not know what to make of today's stories. So weird, so unusual, nearly irrational.

Mia approached with a matcha tea, one americano, a big pitcher of water and one carrot cake with two spoons.

Melo raised her head, fixed her hair behind her ears, and with a big smile on her face said, "Smashing."

The waitress sat close to Melo and said, "Let's share this, it is delicious, it's done every morning by my boss's wife. No, I'm kidding, it's delivered by Jamie, and it is produced by a group of guys who just love baking. They are based in Bermondsey, near Canary wharf."

Melo gave another big smile and said, "That sounds delicious."

The two girls ate eagerly, not saying anything as they caught each other's intermittent gazes, savouring every bit of the cake they could.

Melo put down her spoon, drank a sip of matcha tea and said, "Thank you, that was delicious indeed! We have not been introduced properly. I am Melo Smith, and you are?"

"My name is Catalina Maria Dona Porcel, and I know I look exactly like Mia Wallace from Pulp Fiction, so you can call me Mia like everybody else in London."

Melo shook the hand of her new friend, gazing fixedly into her brown eyes.

"Really nice to know you, Mia. How long have you been working here? Do you know Dr. Elpis?"

"I have been here since 2016. I only know the doctor because of the deal she has with the restaurant. I must come early on Saturday mornings to open for your meeting."

"I know Dr. Elpis is really weird, but she is not a weirdo. Do you know what I mean?"

"Yes. I agree. Dr. Elpis is far from being a weirdo. I never saw her face, but I knew from the beginning that my boss admires her and has been happy to help her with this project. I felt privileged when he asked me to help, even if it meant waking up early every Saturday morning."

"I know what you mean. Today's story was intense and weird, all together. She talked about death and cancer."

"My mother had cancer. But she's fine now, you know. Sometimes it can be hard to talk about it with people, but it's just a part of life."

Melo gazed at Mia in silence.

Mia looked at her mobile. It was time to get ready for the customers.

"I have to get back to work, don't think too much, Melo. Just go enjoy your day."

Melo packed, looked at Mia dearly and said, "Really nice talking with you, I'll see you next Saturday, Ok?"

I will give no deadly medicine to anyone if asked,
nor suggest any such counsel

HIPPOCRATES

Saturday Three

M elo felt her father's hand gently caressing her cheek.
"Wake up, darling Melo, you are going to be late for
your meeting with the doctor."

Melo opened her eyes and grabbed her iPhone. "Oh no, I didn't
hear the alarm."

"Here's a cup of tea, get ready, my beautiful child."

She could not be late. She just couldn't. Melo went straight to
the bathroom, put her clothes on, sipped some tea, and went to
brush her teeth with her Oral-B electric toothbrush and 'clinically
proven' Janina UltraWhite toothpaste. Twenty minutes later, she
was out, walking down Richmond Avenue. Luckily, she got the first
train without delay. And she made it. She arrived at The Mirage at
6:56 am.

Mia was behind the bar, setting up carrot cake slices near a pyramid
of cannoli. On the other side, Melo spotted some lemon cakes and
other tempting delicacies. One day, she'd try one of those.

"Good morning, Melo, your usual matcha tea?" Mia said.

With a slight head movement, Melo nodded and smiled at her
familiar friend. She made her way back to the doctor.

"Good morning, Melo," Elpis began. "It is silliness to live when to
live is torment; and then have we a prescription to die when death
is our physician."

Melo joined in eagerly, "To which Iago replied, 'Ere I would say
I would drown myself for the love of a guinea hen, I would change
my humanity with a baboon.'"

"You know your classics, Melo, I am impressed."

The blogger blushed. It was comforting to have her knowledge
praised by a hooded doctor! The more she got to know the doctor,

the more she felt connected to her. Moments like this made her feel like she was Dr. Elpis' equal, and Melo appreciated it.

"The phrasing of the Hippocratic oath is flawless. 'I will give no deadly medicine to anyone if asked, nor suggest any such counsel.' This is clear cut; assisted suicide should not involve my profession. I am fully aware that some may want the right to die of their own accord. However, doctors should never help with suicide, whatever the motive.

Euthanasia, medical mercy killing, has almost always been forbidden in all society. This ban, in my opinion, has guaranteed the trust between people and doctors.

There have been two periods in human history that have allowed euthanasia to happen. At the time of the third Reich in Germany and today in a few countries.

The first ever law about euthanasia was called 'the law for prevention of hereditary diseased offspring' and was put in place in Germany in 1933, under the directive of Dr. Karl Brandt, who would later work under Hitler. Under the law, doctors selected patients that they deemed incurably sick after medical examination, and then administered a mercy death called, in German, a *gnadentod*.

Now, the word *gnatentod* is hardly even spoken in Germany. It is as if it is banned from speech, as well as from collective memory. In my view, the excess of the Nazi regime started with *the gnadentod*. The law about medical mercy killing paved the way for the murders that the third Reich would be responsible for during the holocaust.

Today, in Holland, Belgium, Luxembourg and in a few American states, euthanasia is authorised by law. You may be wondering about Switzerland. Well, their case is unusual. It does not permit medical euthanasia, and doctors can be condemned if found to practice it. In this country, assisted suicide is authorised but is practiced by non-doctors.

The subject of assisted suicide is, in my view, more societal than medical, more metaphysical than physical. If a person makes the decision to end their life when they know that they are close to death, it is entirely their choice. However, it does not have a place in the rules or regulations of my profession."

Melo interjected, "Don't people have the right to choose how they want to die? Why shouldn't a doctor help them?"

"Here is the difference, Melo. People should be allowed to do what they want with their life unless it is damaging someone else. And ending the life of another human being with drug is just wrong. The world cannot tell people what to do with their lives, but this kind of power has no right to be in the medical field. It is completely incongruent with what we do and what we are there for. One of the issues that has arisen is that people in western society relate medicine, or any medical treatment, to my profession. But we are only allowed to use treatments and medications that are *beneficial to the patient*, and to their health, that is all, we are not drug dealers and should have no power on death. This is very, very important. So today, my dear friend, I have two stories for you."

The blogger gazed at the doctor, at her composed hooded figure and beautiful hands. In Melo's mind, it was a *Hakushiko* mask, the symbol of peace that hangs above her library's fireplace. Melo understood the doctor's desire to wear a hood. She opened her Moleskine notebook, took out one of her pens, positioned one leg over the other, and wrote two simple words at the top of her page: 'Deadly Medicine.'

"I have never told these stories before. But today I will.

A few years ago, I was working in Bicêtre Hospital in le Kremlin Bicêtre on the southern border of Paris. During the French Revolution, this hospital was the very place where Dr. Joseph-Ignace Guillotin was asked by the revolutionaries to find a way to kill people quickly, to kill them cleanly. So he invented the guillotine.

I happened to be working in the exact place where this history evolved when I was called in to help treat a patient that had made an attempt at his own life.

It was the middle of the night. I was asleep in bed when the hospital called me on the telephone. I put my white coat on with the notebook and pen in my right pocket, took my black Littman stethoscope, and left the student room.

It was quite dark and cold outside, and I kept both hands deep in my large pockets as I exited the building and turned left to cross the square. There were cats howling in concert in the pitch-black night. I crossed towards a dim light to enter the underground passage that connected all the departments of the hospital. I left the corridor through a large, heavy, grey door, and walked to the emergency department.

The medical team was already busy, surrounding the patient on the stretcher. The patient was unconscious. The registrar was talking as he assessed the situation and examined the man. I dutifully took my pen and wrote what was said.

Patient unconscious, regular pulse at 90.

'Juno, can you finish the ECG setup, please?'

Regular breathing.

'Elpis, count the breathing.'

Multiple injuries, doubt on multiple vertebral fractures, no apparent active bleeding, ECG in place, sinus heart rate, pulse 90, patient stable.

I wrote and observed.

An IV was set up through one prominent vein on the man's strong, left hand. Once his vitals were stable and all his fractures were securely maintained that we were sure he was not bleeding, the registrar ordered, 'Elpis, stay with the patient please, keep an eye on him. Always look at this screen, the infusion line, and count his breathing, all right? You will be alright, Elpis.'

The registrar left and I escorted the patient to the scanner centre, walking by his side.

Following this observation mission, another case required my attention, and another one, etc, etc. And life went on as usual. Until a few months later.

I was in the orthopaedic ward with a fellow classmate of mine. He had asked me for some notes from a lecture that he had missed the day before. I proudly pulled the bunch of papers from my satchel and handed them over to him. He thanked me kindly, and then pointed to a young man with dark, curly hair in a wheelchair at the end of the corridor and said, 'Look at this guy in the wheelchair, he jumped from a bridge because of a girl! She left him and he decided to jump to his death!'

I remembered. I recognised the man from that night a few months ago. This was the boy who had been brought to the hospital in critical condition with multiple severe injuries. I had no idea that it was self-inflicted. I had assumed he had been in a car crash, or some horrific accident had occurred. But to learn that this man had tried to take his own life, and then to see him sitting there laughing, I couldn't decide what to feel first. I was heartbroken to learn that he had wanted to die, but reassured that he had now found the ability to feel joy again. It was the first time I had faced the idea of suicide outside of the classroom. It's one of the first things we are taught as doctors, to detect whether someone is a danger to themselves. We have a list of questions and, also, signs that we look for to diagnose potential depression and suicidal risk. But this was the first time I had ever seen it in action.

I remember I was on shift the night he came. I had no idea this was an attempted suicide case, and I didn't know he survived. It was great to see him laughing.

I asked my friend, 'What is his current situation?'

'He still has a broken vertebra; he sadly won't walk again. But his brain has fully recovered, and he will have no long-term effects. He regained his consciousness two weeks after the coma.'

Dearest Melo, this man had wanted to die. He thought he could not take life anymore; he thought his heartbreak was incurable. But, a few months later, he was joking with some nurses, and making a fool of himself. He seemed chatty and happy. I remember passing by and saying hello to all, keeping an appropriate distance, with a feeling of amazement in my mind.

There will always be people that are facing depression, and that believe in their heart they want to leave. But no matter how an individual may be feeling, we know, my profession and I, that people are capable of great strength, and my job as a doctor is to help them get towards the path of that inner strength. My point was proven here. Although in a moment, this man *a frolé la mort*, he was nearly touching death, but because we were able to save him, he got another chance. This is the noble part of my profession."

Melo was well experienced in meeting with Dr. Elpis. She had caught on to the stories' flow and go, and when a narrative had ended. She looked at Elpis, "I never thought about the medical profession much before meeting you, Elpis. But I must admit, I find it's always on my mind now. I am becoming more and more aware of the necessity of a rulebook, of a guideline to follow morally. I have a lot of respect for what you do, Doctor."

"Melo, medical care is at the same level as justice. In many ways, they are the same. If we do not have a moral code in law, we become inhuman. If we do not have a moral code in medicine, we become inhuman too.

The thing I find difficult in following any code in society is that we, as human beings, are complex and emotional. Our feelings can often take jurisdiction over our actions. Thinking rationally when such emotions as love and hate are involved can get very tricky.

For a professional in the fleeting moment, I have only two things that I need. My learned skill and the oath. Nothing else is at play. Regardless of whether the patient I am treating is a stranger, like the man in the wheelchair, or someone that I love, the process is the same.

Years ago, my mother Paulette died at the too-young age of sixty-two. A malignant melanoma invaded her tiny, still young, strong and beautiful body. The cancer won the unfair battle, invading her lungs and brain in a matter of days.

My mother was a survivor. She had recovered from two near-death experiences before the last one which caught up to her.

Paulette was born prematurely in 1929 and was kept in a shoe box for the first few weeks of her life, but she survived. Born to a poor family in Normandy, my mother's life was only about survival, and she did it better than anyone. At thirteen, she was diagnosed with the disease diphtheria, known at the time as a child killer. Although a vaccine had already been created in 1926 against this disease, my mother did not have access to it. But still, she survived. She went on to have nine children, but lost one son, Vivien at thirteen. My father, her husband, suffered from early-onset dementia, leaving her in charge of the family and the carpenter's business at the age of thirty-seven. If my mother knew how to do anything, it was to survive.

The final act of Paulette's life started following an excision and removal of a cyst on the side of her knee. When her consultant dermatologist found out that she had a doctor in the family, he called the doctor, me, directly.

'Elpis, this is Doctor Moreau, I'm calling about your mother. I am sorry to tell you that the cyst is actually a metastasis of a malignant melanoma. Sadly, the scans have revealed further lesions in the lung and brain. I am sorry, Elpis, there is no hope.'

I was shocked, took a seat, and tried to reconcile my own feelings. I remember exactly where I was. At this point I was placed in a psychiatric ward in Brest, Brittany. Rare, shouted words were breaking the clinical silence, patients were smoking in the communal room, not speaking to anyone. I was on shift when I got the call.

'Doctor, what should we do?' I asked.

'I am sorry, but not much can be done. We have just started a trial with Interferon, an immune modulator, which may help. In view of the extent of your mother's disease, it is unlikely it would work though, but one cannot be sure. Elpis, should I inform your mother of the prognosis, propose getting her involved in the trial, or should we limit our work to palliative care without telling her?'

I felt the first signs of fainting as I began to perspire profusely. I held onto the back of the chair to avoid collapsing but managed to pronounce a few words.

'Let me talk to my brothers and sisters.'

'I understand, call me next week before my next appointment with your mother.'

My family met the next day. I informed everyone. A conclusion was reached. The doctor should tell the whole truth to our mother, who should decide for herself. We all guessed that it was what our mother would want.

A few days later, I accompanied Paulette to her next appointment. She was told by the consultant that the prognosis was very poor with the cancer already spreading to her lungs. He walked her through everything that we knew and proposed the options. I remember being impressed with my mother's aura, she was calm and rational. She did not even ask if she would be cured, she just replied, 'We should try then.'

I wanted to hold my mother, to feel her skin, to cry in her arms. But I did not, I was baffled by her matter-of-factness, and in awe of the older and experienced human being my mother was! There was a kind of serenity, a surrender to nothing less than a death sentence mixed with the want to live.

Sadly, the brain metastasis developed very quickly damaging the brain functions one by one. Half of her visual field went. A few weeks later, her coordination was affected, making it impossible to hold a spoon, and then to walk. Next her speech slurred and finally continence disappeared, an initial sign that death was coming, and it did, forty-eight hours later.

At this point, my mother was being looked after by my sister in her home in Lannion, seventy kilometres from Brest, and my medical practice. I remember calling my sister to check in, and she told me that our mother was sleeping and could not be woken up. I understood immediately and asked my colleague to take over the care of my patients for the next few days. I drove, listening to France Culture, my preferred French radio station. I remember driving in the rain the entire way, trying not to think about what was to come. When I arrived, my sister welcomed me in silence. Our mother was unconscious. The family doctor had left some injectable morphine and aspiration equipment. We called the rest of the family, and everyone came to say goodbye.

I recall sitting on the right side of my mother who was breathing heavily. She began vomiting a very dark sticky liquid, even though she remained unconscious. The noise and the dark vomit were a lot for all of us to take in, but I stayed strong and professional and treated my mother exactly as I would a patient in the hospital, guided by my skills and the oath. I skilfully aspirated the terrible charcoal-black vomit and managed to avoid any spillage; cleanliness was maintained till the very end. I injected morphine regularly, with the purpose of reducing her suffering. I was fully conscious that morphine was, in a way, accelerating the process towards death, and possibly robbing my mother of more minutes or even hours on Earth. However, my only purpose was to preserve her dignity in the face of death.

I knew that I did not have the power to give her back her life, but I did know that I could care for her till the end. And I did.

My mother died early in the morning, surrounded by all her family.

I do not recall the actual moment of death, or the moments that followed. I erased it from my mind in the mourning process. But I remember driving that afternoon to the nearby town in Lannion, passing by the old half-timbered and slate-clad houses with my eldest sister.

We parked the car and walked in silence down the street named Rue des Chapeliers, then crossed the square named Place du Marhallac'h towards the west side and the tower of Saint-Jean-du-Baly. We then took the first right to the street named, then turn right to the street called Rue de Saint Malo. The day was the Saturday before Christmas. The streets were crowded with noisy and joyful people: children and families shopping, and ladies chatting on the pavement with their many different-coloured shopping bags. The shop windows were illuminated with beautiful Christmas displays. The whole scene was so illusory for me and my sister, who just a few hours ago, had assisted our mother through her last day on Earth. It was eerie, all of this Christmas frenzy. The colours were too vibrant, the noises distorted and aggressively loud. However, we had to do what we came here for, and we kept silent, walking with a determined pace through the joyful crowd. We finally arrived at our destination, a shop well-known for its lace clothing and Christian jewellery. We agreed promptly and bought a pure cotton, white nightdress with delicate lace and very thin nacre buttons, along with a rosary with a finely carved, silver crucifix, and wooden pearls. We agreed that our mother would have liked them.

Back home, we carefully put the white lace dress on my mother and buttoned up the sleeves around her smooth, dead wrists. We placed the rosary between her already rigid fingers and interlocked her hands into a prayer position on her chest. We turned the rosary's crucifix outwards, with Jesus Christ facing up.

My mother was ready, her friends and family would visit her and mourn. She would be buried five days later.

I could not stay; I had to go back to Brest to work the following day. But on my way back home, I drove through my village, and passed by the church from my childhood. I felt the need to go back to my roots that day. I wanted to see the gargoyles, the apocalyptic dragons with the *ankou* I loved so much.

I passed by the church with the song *Wish you were here* on the tape player. As the sound of David Gilmour's voice crept through my speakers, I finally cried. Warm, salty tears poured down my cheeks and lips. I sobbed and howled from my heart, as if something was releasing from deep inside me. I cried loudly, free from onlookers, and free from my doctor status. I cried until I reached my home in Brest.

And life carried on as it always does.

Paulette died with dignity. I helped my own mother on the journey to meet death, in the same way I have and would with any patient of mine. All I needed was the oath and respect for humanity.

The doctor sited: '*I will give no deadly medicine to anyone if asked, nor suggest any such counsel.*'"

Melo watched the hooded doctor as she brought her ring-filled hands to her face beneath her hood. Her chest rose and fell faster than usual. Melo could tell she was hurt, maybe even crying. She did not know what to say or do. She wished she could see the doctor's eyes, but she knew she never would. She waited and watched, waited and watched. The light around them seemed to be getting dimmer, as if reality was pulsating. Melo felt inadequate. She tried to think of what would console Elpis, she knew words would not be enough. She wished she had her guitar so she could play something soothing. She remembered Elpis' dream she had with Hippocrates and how he played his kithara for her, and an idea sprung to mind. She began searching her phone for the sounds of the kithara, and when she stumbled on one that was recalling ancient Greek sounds, she knew it was the one. Melo pressed play on her phone and placed the music on the table between the doctor and her.

The doctor's body immediately went still, almost as if she was a statue. She slowly moved her neck forward, about to reveal her face from below her hood, but stopped herself before she could. The doctor bowed her head lower once again.

Melo wished to see the doctor's face but knew it would break the code that they had created amongst themselves. Melo felt close to the doctor, even though she could not see her or touch her. Still, she felt that she knew the human being she was, and she felt known in return. And then, like a magic trick, Mia appeared.

"Can I get you guys anything?"

Elpis finally spoke. "No thank you. It is time for me to go. Thank you for the music, Melo, I'll always remember that."

"You're welcome, Doctor Elpis. Thank you too."

Elpis left, and the girls were left behind.

▲

That night, Melo went straight to visit her father in his study. The man was at his desk, studying an A3 document filled with emojis. He was working on the past, current and future linguistic consequences of the use of the Japanese characters in the English language. He had to finish a paper before the end of the month.

Melo grabbed her special wooden stool with its oriental tapestry cover and brought it next to her father's desk to sit with him. She rested her right hand on his shoulder and leaned her head on his left side. She watched as he studied the document before him.

Melo asked, "Daddy, were Granddad's hands cold and smooth when he died?"

After a few minutes of silence, the man replied.

"Yes indeed, I remember it well. His skin was very smooth. It was cold too."

Melo had never really spoken with her father about her granddad's death. He had been gone for over twenty years before she was born. She'd only heard stories and regretted never having asked more about him and what he was like.

"Daddy, can you tell me more about your father?"

"Okay, my dear. Why don't you get two cups of tea started, and I'll finish up my work?"

Melo eagerly left the library and went to the kitchen to get two cups of tea and a slice of carrot cake. She placed them on a tray and walked back to the library to see her dad sitting on the sofa, opposite the wall with the *Hakushiko* mask. She put the tray on the table on the right-hand side. Her father bent down and grabbed a big photo album from the drawer under the table. He placed it on the table and opened it to one of the middle pages. He pointed to one of the photos.

"This is him and I before I went to university."

He looked very old to Melo.

"Your grandfather was very sick. I always knew him as a sick person. Now, we would say he had PTSD, but he was never able to integrate in society when he returned, and he was also constantly physically battling something. There was always a doctor coming to visit him and fix some ailment. He was very discreet, and he never spoke about his experiences with any of us. He always said the phrase "I have already died". He was very interested in linguistics though; he was the one who inspired me. His dad had worked in publishing.

The love of the books and words has long been in our family. I know he would have really loved your work."

The two sat together and flipped through the family photo book for a long while. In every photo, Melo's grandfather looked detached from the life he was pictured living. She had empathy for her father's upbringing. She realised it was vastly different from how she was raised. The two finished their tea and shared the carrot cake, and closed the night early. Both needed rest.

I will not give to a woman a pessary
to produce abortion

HIPPOCRATES

Saturday Four

Melo worked a lot that week. She had to finish one post for the blog, and the night before she had a studio practice with her band. The session was intense, and on that occasion, she stayed with everyone for a drink. Brian, the drummer, bought her a Coca-Cola and sat silently by her side. They did not talk, just listened to the others and laughed at the jokes. Melo did not think about death or Elpis' stories.

Melo woke up that Saturday morning fatigued, but she got up anyway. She got dressed listening to some music and left the house as usual, heading for her now routine tube ride.

As she walked through Soho, Melo listened to *Stairway To Heaven* by Led Zeppelin with her Bose earphones. She wondered what Elpis did in her free time and what kind of life she lived outside of The Mirage.

She arrived at the restaurant at 6:58 am and found Elpis sitting quietly surrounded by a dim light. It almost looked like she had a halo around her hood.

Mia said loudly, "Good Morning! I'll bring your matcha tea right over."

Melo turned her head and acknowledged the offer with a wink from behind her curls.

"Good morning, Melo."

"Good morning, Doctor."

As usual, Dr. Elpis opened today's subject without any small talk or even comment on what had happened last week.

"In 2006, a whale appeared in the Thames River, just near the parliament building and Big Ben. Her normal habitat was supposed to be around the coasts in the far north of Scotland, Northern Ireland

and in the seas around the Arctic Ocean, far from the Thames.

Apparently, the animal had taken a wrong turn. Many experts assumed that while swimming down the east coast and wanting to go to the west to join her family, she turned into the Thames Estuary, rather than where she should have turned miles further south in the Channel. She just took a wrong turn.

I called the whale Mocha Dick from the day she arrived. That was the name of the real-life albino whale that inspired the book Moby Dick.

I watched the story unfold from my television while many Londoners were already gathering on the riverbanks to try to spot the animal. The reporter said that rescuers had been called. After hours of swimming hopelessly in the Thames, the poor thing became beached. The rescue team of experts, already on watch, quickly moved the animal onto an inflatable pontoon, keeping Mocha Dick in water with her blowhole above the surface. The experts assessed her state of health, the prognosis, and their actual chance of saving the animal. Under the eyes of all Londoners, the scientists and marine mammal experts performed ultrasounds, blood tests, and assessed the animal's breathing and general presentation. The process was nearly identical to the treatment of a person.

The plan was to transfer the animal from the pontoon to a deep-sea ship. The experts first needed to assess Mocha Dick's vital signs before planning anything. However, the condition of the whale deteriorated, and sadly the animal died from convulsions around 7 pm on the 21st of January 2006.

Thousands of Londoners were packed along the river, devastated by Mocha Dick's death; they had become collectively attached to her in a single instant. No one had to convince them otherwise. The subsequent autopsy revealed that the animal had sustained many injuries and was at that point in time suffering from kidney failure, which certainly precipitated her death. While experts attempted to make sense of how the whale ended up there, it didn't matter in any way in the effort to save her. The people watching didn't want to know why she was there, but how we were going to get her back to safety in the wild.

While Mocha Dick was unable to be saved, we as a human race were still able to care for the animal and have empathy with no restraint. It was never something anyone tried to gain power over. We just trusted the experts.

But what happens when a human being takes a wrong turn in their life? How do we, as a society react?

When I was twenty-three years old, I went to the Rodin Museum in Paris, Rue de Varenne, five minutes' walk from the tomb of Napoleon in the Pantheon. I was strolling through the majestic building when I encountered the bust called 'La Chatelaine'. It was discreetly positioned in the stairway of the grand house. Yet the artwork caught my attention at first sight. It was both unusually feminine and powerful. I looked closer and read that it was made by a woman named Camille Claudel. While most of the work highlighted and at the forefront of exhibits was Rodin's artwork, intermixed were the sculptures of Claudel. I had to hunt to find them, as they were often hidden in discreet places, hiding behind the work of the man.

Later on, while I was going through a bookstore in the Quartier Latin, I stumbled upon this name once more: Camille Claudel. I began reading. She was a student of Rodin and had an affair with him, and that was the wrong turn. I read that some of Rodin's sculptures were made by four hands, the hands of Auguste Rodin working in concert with Camille Claudel's.

I understood, the woman was beautiful, full of life, gifted and a hard worker.

Rodin and Camille had a love affair for more than ten years while they were working together. During this time, Claudel made magnificent work, but she did not sell much in comparison to her teacher. Women's art had no demand in society, it was undervalued. She had no way of becoming an independent artist.

However, one wrong turn and the young artist got pregnant. As an unmarried woman, a daughter of a French bourgeoise Catholic family, and the mistress of a famous artist, she had no option but to abort. It is even likely that she was forced to do so.

Following Camille's unwanted pregnancy, she was rejected by her lover and shut away from society, as well as her own family. Following the event, the subsequent denial of motherhood, the breakdown of her relationship, and the loss of her position as an artist, she suffered from severe depression. Of course, she did! I would have too!

At the height of her depression, she showed up outside Rodin's home, yelling her pain. His response was to contact her family and ask them to deal with her behaviour. Deeply ashamed of her and her actions, her mother sectioned her to a psychiatric hospital under the diagnosis of 'hysteria.' Women were not allowed to be depressed, they were only allowed to be crazy. She would live in that hospital for the next thirty years until her ultimate death, despite doctors' reports of good mental health and the continuous plea from her loyal British friend Jesse Lipscomb—a fellow student of Rodin—for her to be discharged from the hospital. Camille would be buried anonymously in the communal tomb of the town with the other destitute.

Camille Claudel's destiny is one poignant example of how the life of a woman can be affected by the opinions and beliefs of others. It is the story of the abandonment of a woman not only by her lover, but also by her family and the whole of society following an abortion.

Unfortunately, and rather shamefully for our humanity, many other women have the same story to tell, across generations and all around the globe. In the western world, we have a way to use the mistakes that we are all capable of as a means to gain power, especially politically. When it comes to an animal who takes a wrong turn, there is no power to be gained. So people respond quickly and positively, immediately feeling empathy for the animal and the mistake it has made. Whereas with the life of a woman, there is plenty of power to be gained. Such is the story of Camille's tragic life. We treat people as collateral damage.

Today, some women have physical suffering with complications from unsafe abortions, such as punctures of the uterus or vagina or other severe injury: fistulas, septicaemia and tetanus. Many women still die within the few weeks following an unsafe abortion.

Even now, more than a hundred years after Camille's abortion—despite medical advances—we have many women around the world still suffering in mind and body, especially in countries at war. Today, unwanted pregnancies are weaponised by governments and their policies. The so-called Global Gag Ban is a ban set up by the United States towards charities that work in these war-torn countries. The ban has existed on and off for many years and, when in place, means that any charity working abroad and funded by American people or businesses are not allowed to offer medical abortions to the women that they were helping.

When Donald Trump was elected, one of the first things he did was put this ban back in place.

France, Germany and Britain stay on the side of the United States, while Norway, Sweden and the Netherlands joined a coalition of human rights groups in calling on the US to lift its abortion ban on aid for women raped in war as a matter of compliance with the Geneva Convention. Nevertheless, the ban is still in action and there to stay despite being inhuman and a disgraceful aggravation of rape as an instrument of war! And it is certain that Hippocrates would be shocked on the way global politics is interfering with the relationship between physicians and patients, even though the oath stipulates '*I will not give to a woman a pessary to produce abortion.*'

In the 5th century BC, at the time of Hippocrates, the attempted abortions were critically harmful to not only the baby, but the women. So regardless of whether someone needed it or not, they would be severely damaged. This line in the oath was to protect first and foremost women's health.

Now, with the advancements of medicine, we know not only how a baby develops but also how to perform a safe abortion to protect women's lives when morally applicable.

What science knows for certain is that in human pregnancies, a baby is an embryo until week eleven, and not yet a complete little human being. The embryonic period is all about the formation of systems in the body. At week twelve, this process is achieved and the baby's foundation and framework is there, with one brain, one heart beating, two lungs, two kidneys, one liver, four limbs, ten fingers, ten toes, a tongue, a nose, etc, etc.

The foetal state, the period when the baby is a full human being, starts at twelve weeks and then it is all about growth and development of the fully formed human being. That is why France and many other countries adopted the twelve week limit for legal abortion.

In the UK today, the ban does not affect us. Abortion is free and available to all in this country, both immigrants and UK citizens. However, activists demonstrate their hate for abortion. Both extremes are incorrect and dangerous. You cannot just have all abortion, or no abortion. It is a private decision. These people that protest are for their own opinions, not the reality of the situation. Hippocrates would have described both extremes as ferocious, barbaric and cruel. Unfortunately, these individuals are here to stay.

When I trained as a doctor in the 1980s, abortion was already legal in France. It had been since 1975. I have always worked with the law on the side of safe abortion, but I believe there are a set of circumstances that determine whether it is moral or immoral. It does not take religion to determine whether something is moral, it takes common sense and communication without judgement.

Now, let me tell you about one family I looked after many years ago in Brest, Brittany.

Once, a pack of bottlenose whales were swimming north-west off the coast of the city, which was once a penal colony where Victor Hugo decided to set Jean Valjean's prison sentence in his book *Les Miserables*.

A busy day ahead. After reading a few letters, reports and results, I was ready to begin a shift at my practice. I walked into the waiting room and called for my first patient, Madame Ginette Cadiou.

'*Docteur, je ne me sens pas bien.* I feel sick, especially in the morning.'

'How long have you been feeling like this?' I said.

'For about two weeks. At first, I thought I had eaten something bad, but I did not get any diarrhoea or stomach pain. I am just sick. My mother had gallbladder surgery a few years ago. Doctor, do you think that's what this could be?'

I then asked Ginette to undress and lie down on the examining couch.

The woman was a young mother of two little girls. She was a blonde with fair skin and faint freckles on her cheeks ready to flare up at the first rays of sunshine. She was wearing discreet white underwear, a gold crucifix she may have had since her baptism, and on her fingers were two rings: one was her wedding ring and the other was an old, antique ring possibly from her grandmother.

I examined her in silence and thought, she looked healthy. No noticeable pallor, temperature at 37.5, pulse at 90, blood pressure low at 90/60. The chest and abdomen examinations were both reassuring. I examined her and thought, *the woman is pregnant!*

I told her she could get dressed, and that I needed a urine sample. I gave her a 60 ml container. Ginette had been my patient for several years. She knew where to go and left my office for the bathroom without question. She came back in a few minutes and handed over the container with the pale-yellow liquid, then sat at the desk.

I inspected and put the container on the table for a specimen examination. I dipped two devices into the urine, one for biochemistry and one for pregnancy testing. Then I removed one of them after 10 seconds to lay it flat on a dry tissue on the table. I then joined the young patient for discussion.

'Mrs. Cadiou, when was your last period?'

'Oh, I cannot remember, let me think about it. Euh, I think that was around the first of March, the Sunday my in-laws came from Paris.'

'So, that was ten weeks ago. You may be pregnant, you know.'

'That is not possible, Doctor. My two girls were conceived with IVF, don't you remember? I can't be pregnant just like that.'

I did not reply but got up and went to the table, checked the strip still in the urine and looked at the testing device. The two red lines were there. Ginette was pregnant. I came back to my chair with a big smile on my face and said,

'The pregnancy test is positive. Nature is sometimes unpredictable but wonderful.'

'What? Are you sure, Doctor? But, how did this happen? What am I going to do? I need to talk to my husband.' She was obviously at a loss and asked, 'Doctor, what is the limit date for abortion please?'

I was shocked but kept my countenance steady. A few minutes before, I'd been so happy, as I always am when I diagnose pregnancy! How could a mother of two, a woman who went through several IVF treatments, think, even for an instant, of getting rid of this unexpected pregnancy? How could she?

However, I kept calm and professional, kept my kind voice, and informed the patient as required, 'Mrs. Cadiou, the legal limit is twelve weeks. You have time to think. Go back home, talk to your husband and come back to me next week.' I wanted to say, 'Hang on, how can you think of abortion, how can you stop the wonder of life?' But I would never say that. I have to be professional, caring, and informative, without any opinion or prejudice whatsoever. Ginette left, and I got ready for the other patients of the day. Time passed, and five days later, the mother of two and her husband came back to see me as planned.

I welcomed the couple, a bit sad that I might have to arrange an abortion for a child who may be coming at the wrong time in these people's lives. Deep inside, I felt the situation was a bit unfair and selfish. But I was a doctor who mustn't be governed by my own feelings, ever.

Both husband and wife sat down. Mr. Cadiou said, 'We have done another test at home, it's positive. We are surprised though, as we were told we could not have children naturally.'

'These things happen,' I replied.

His wife was silent, her face looking towards the floor.

'Mrs. Cadiou, how do you feel?'

'I feel sick every morning, and so tired, Doctor. Cleo, our eldest

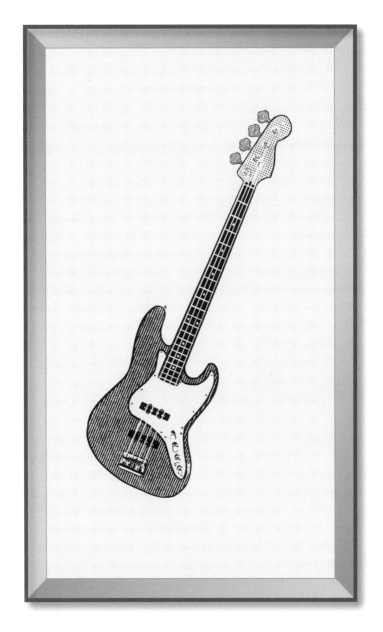

daughter, is asking why.'

'Have you told her?' I asked.

Her husband replied, 'Doctor, this situation is so unexpected.'

'I know, life is like that sometimes.'

'Yes, Doctor,' Ginette said. 'Are you sure that's it? I'm pregnant?'

I know this behaviour well. People repeat themselves in states of disbelief. They need reassurance and repeating things help.

'Yes, Mrs. Cadiou, you are pregnant. What do you want to do?'

A silence settled in the room, I waited quietly and cautiously. I felt the mixed feelings of husband and wife. I knew what had happened and I just focused my mind on the knowledge of the wonder of life.

I knew the whole human story, its timing, lifestyle, emotion and biology. I knew. A few weeks before husband and wife had made love and one of the spermatozoa from the multitude had made it!

On that very day, the family's two daughters had finally been sleeping. The couple went to bed, exhausted. Their two bodies drew closer, hands and lips touching. Husband and wife made love, as they had done many times before and after. Ginette felt the bodily effects of the neurotransmitters' apocalyptic storm called orgasm. The dopamine flowed in along with noradrenaline, adrenaline, testosterone, and the precious oxytocin. Thereafter, her husband experienced the identical phenomenon, with a rush of the same amount of dopamine, adrenaline, noradrenaline, more of testosterone but less oxytocin. The two bodies relaxed, the two human beings felt love for and contentment in each other, hands and legs intertwined, both bodies finding their foetal position, two bodies embedded in each other's. Two bodies, one couple and love. Meanwhile, the sperm was flowing in both directions, between Ginette's warm legs and up to her womb. Her husband's hand rested on her beautiful tummy—and in the unknown, in the inside of that very tummy, millions of spermatozoa rushed up Ginette's relaxed vagina towards their desired destination, the human's womb. From thousands of the ejaculated millions, the strongest and the fittest went through the cervix. A few made it and reached the womb of the woman, but only one will go beyond.

And on that very day, one single egg was there in all its glory, its size a thousand times the size of the one chosen spermatozoon. It was there, at the very moment, one unique spermatozoon made it.

Both husband and wife were by now in their individual dream worlds. One single male gamete, the quickest and the fittest spermatozoa, penetrated the outer jelly coat of Ginette's majestic egg. Its acrosome produced enzymes which allowed it to burrow through the coat of the egg. Its plasma then fused with the egg's membrane, its head disconnected from its flagellum and then, and then, over a few days, the fertilised egg travelled gently down the fallopian tube to reach the uterus where it would transform itself into a human baby.

Six days later, husband and wife were eating with their two daughters, all talking and laughing when human chorionic gonadotrophin production kicked off to help the egg with its nutritious settlement in the uterus, where it shall stay for the next nine months or so.

Ginette got pregnant!

But I supposed the family had their life organised and planned for two children and not three. There were only three bedrooms in their home, the car was a small, cherry-red Renaud 5. There were holidays planned for four of them in nine months' time. This event, the human's conception, even with all its glory, was just so unplanned. It was a wrong turn in their life.

Finally, Ginette broke the silence and asked me, 'Can you refer me for an ultrasound, just to check?'

'Of course.' I filled in the form, called the radiology centre and booked her an appointment.

The couple did not come back to me. Rather, I received three consecutive letters from an obstetrician consultant reporting the good health of the mother and baby to be. They decided not to abort in the end.

A few months passed, and I was busy with many other various issues.

Then one day, as some bottlenose whales swam together in the far distant sea, a little boy named Clement was born.

Life is like that, sometimes.

I had the privilege to be called to see Clement for his first examination before mother and child could leave the hospital. I was so happy, I cannot tell you, so happy. And so was the family. They were on top of the moon with their newborn. This was one of the great joys of my profession which is no more unfortunately: going to the hospital and talking to the parents, examining the newborn, and checking that all the reflexes were already there! My favourite thing was to check is the baby's grip. I put my finger in the newborn's palm and watch as they grip back and walk. Did you know that if you put a finger in both palms of a newborn, the grip is instinctual and so strong that if you lifted the baby up, he or she would not let go and start walking. That is the strength and human instinct of a newborn baby.

My work done, I said goodbye, and with all my heart, I wished a long life to Baby Clement!

You see, Melo, when it comes to the discussion of abortion, there is no one answer. There are only the circumstances that surround the choice. That is what I, as a doctor, look at when I am confronted with these situations.

What I wish to see in the world is a place where communication between professionals and the people are free flowing and open and get back in the privacy. We do not need politicians, industries, or lawyers to deal with medical situations, and as such it does not need to veer outside our spaces and the intimacy of that space.

The villain in the Claudel story was the society that judged and destroyed a promising woman and let her be carted away to an insane asylum based on a single mistake that was mutually committed by both her and Rodin.

With the family in Brest, they only decided with the doctor. It was no one else's choice or business. They decided for themselves without society's prejudice or knowledge.

Now, as a modern society, we have medical abortion and people who are able to make their own choices for their health. We do not need input from anyone else. And I know Hippocrates would have agreed—and been amazed—knowing what we know now."

Melo stayed silent. No word uttered. She was in awe of the meeting that day. Never before had she seen such a complicated human debate broken down to such common sense and wisdom. It was today that Melo knew she was meant to be there to hear the doctor's stories. She was beginning to understand fully why the doctor had been so adamant about finding a digital native to share these stories. It was a work of intergenerational transmission.

As the doctor left as she always does, Melo packed up her black notebook and three pens and knew there was work to be done.

*With purity and with holiness I will pass my life
and practise my Art*

HIPPOCRATES

Saturday Five

The night before, Melo had stayed up late. She'd wanted to know more about hormones and anatomy and googled sites of all kinds, getting carried away and falling asleep in front of the screen.

At 5.30 am, Melo's iPhone broke into the ripples tone, the melodic sound she had chosen from Apple's pre-programmed list. She opened her eyes but did not move from the foetal position. She had fallen asleep with her clothes on the night before and awoke with pins and needles in her thighs from the tightly kept jeans she was wearing.

She looked over to her still open laptop screen to find it was pitch black.

Her room still smelled like fresh paint from the new coat that was added late last month. Melo had wanted a change and asked her parents. She wanted her room painted in black, but her mother talked her into something less dreary. They agreed on a Midlake grey. She didn't have time to put up posters yet, but she did hang her Yamaha four string bass guitar on the wall opposite her bed.

Melo's hand reached for her phone. In a hurry, she stood up but nearly fell from her jeans down to her legs. In a snake-like movement, the girl pulled down her jeans and pants, and with one foot took it all off. She plugged in the nearly dead laptop and then went to the bathroom.

Melo began to brush her teeth and, without thinking, gently brought her free hand to her stomach, and tenderly covered her umbilicus with the tip of her thumb. She lightly spread her hand over her body, letting her middle finger fiddle with one of her soft golden curls there, down below.

It was nice and warm. The young woman felt the natural heat of her body and imagined she was holding her womb. Melo liked it. In her mind, the doctor's words echoed along with the images she had looked up the night before while researching: the uterus with its triangular shape and something like two ears at the top, reminding Melo of her Baby Yoda. The young woman winked at the mirror to that thought. There was no time to waste, she had to get ready.

She went back to her bedroom and eagerly reached the cupboard to take out her brand-new cycling gear. It was a special day indeed. Melo was to cycle to her rendezvous with the doctor. Her parents had finally agreed to it. The young woman felt delighted and full of joy. She was impatient to listen to another story. Melo kept thinking about the way Elpis described the creation process, how we've all come to be. She wanted more of this.

The gear was easy to put on, it fit her perfectly around her svelte legs and tiny waist. In three swift movements, she arranged her hair and was ready to go. Before leaving, Melo went to the kitchen to show off and kiss her parents goodbye. Lifting their heads in concert, mother and father gazed at her and both gave approving smiles. Melo went to kiss her father on his bald head, and her mother on the cheek already positioned for the goodbye kiss.

"Have fun, Melo."

"I should be back at nine," she said, to which her father murmured, "Remember, Melo, I'm leaving for Japan today. I'll be back next week."

"I remember. Good luck with the conference and have fun!"

Father and mother went back to reading the weekend newspapers in the silent kitchen, with only the tick of the Victorian clock for company.

Out of the door, Melo tightened the ratchet of her helmet, threw one leg over her bike, and rode off. Leaving Richmond, Melo reached the Thames path in an instant. The river was bordered by grand mansions and the water was still that day. As she rode, the air ran through the holes in her helmet, the breeze was crisp but refreshing. When she passed Putney Bridge, Mocha Dick came to mind. She wondered how far she was from where the whale had lost its way. There were at least twenty cormorants along the river that morning, just on one barge, all together like a team. Some were standing and others were immobile, their wings spread letting the air come through, like they were having a rest. As Melo looked at them, she realised they must be feeling the same sensation as her, the wind comforting their bodies this beautiful morning. She spotted one of these birds, all alone and isolated, laying on its side. In the ignorance of the others, this bird was not helped. These animals were not like her kind, she thought. No other cormorant was around this sad one. And for sure, these animals would not have cared for Mocha Dick. Humans help other species but also each other when they are hurt, or at least, are supposed to.

Still cycling, thinking and imagining, the blogger crossed Chelsea, up through Kensington to Hyde Park. It was quiet, with no traffic, so it was an easy cycling trip. During her descent to Piccadilly Street, Melo spotted the closed Royal Academy gates. They looked much bigger than usual without the crowd. The dragons of the apocalypse were visible and imposing, Melo thought.

She arrived at her destination at 6.50 am and parked her bicycle opposite The Mirage.

Mia was outside, setting up tables. "Hi, good morning. Nice bike, lucky you."

"Thank you. Hackney Cycles made it specially for me and according to my specifications. I love it. Look at the Nologo wheels, wicked, no? And the light frame, and the bullhorn handlebars. I just like the design and it gets good traction on the street! And look, Mia, my name is on the frame!"

"Really nice. This must have cost a fortune!"

"Not at all, only two hundred with a one-year guarantee and free service. My dad bought it for me. You know he does everything to push me away from my laptop!"

"That's not bad." Mia got closer to the bike and, with an ironic smile, said, "Hey, Melo, you've locked your bike to a drainpipe! This bike you love so much will be gone in thirty minutes. Lock it to the railing just there, it's much safer."

Mia was now convinced that Melo was a rich kid without any common sense. But she liked her anyway. She felt a draw towards this blonde girl and thought they could really be friends if they had the opportunity to speak alone. Decisively, she took the lock from Melo's hand and proceeded with the safer option, locking both the front wheel and the frame to the railing. Melo stood still and watched as Mia fixed up her bike.

Mia looked up at Melo, and said dryly with a smile, "I'll bring your matcha tea." Melo laughed, and the two side by side entered The Mirage side by side.

At the sight of the doctor at the back of the room, the joy of the early morning came back to her. With no hesitation, she walked back, sat down, and with a decisive tone, the blogger said, "Good morning, Dr. Elpis."

"Good morning, Melo. I like your cycling gear. Slate grey stripes on a mellow yellow design, very special. It suits your golden curls."

"Oh, thank you. My father bought it for me. He wanted me to be visible all the time. Do you want to come outside and have a look at the bike?"

"Not now, Melo, later maybe. How was the travel from home?"

Would Dr. Elpis ever leave her chair? Would Melo ever see the doctor outside of The Mirage? She doubted it and just said,

"Quite good, actually. My home is in Richmond, and I rode along the Thames to come in. There was not much traffic, and I saw some arrogant cormorants on a barge."

"Arrogant cormorants—Melo, you are funny. I like your choice of words."

"My dad is a linguist and my mother a lawyer. Words are very important in our family."

"I suppose your father chose your name 'Melo', the Greek root for melody. Is that correct?"

The blogger hesitated and then said, "Dad chose my name, that's true, but after the French film *Melo*. He said the film was just beautiful. In any case, I like my name."

"I like it too, and I must admit, it suits you perfectly. Let's begin, shall we?"

While my ancestors were helped by the idea of God and holiness, I was not. I know that holiness exists for many and needs to be respected, whatever the form or shape it has. It can be religion, animist beliefs, metaphysics or pure spirituality away from any religion. The oath means the sacrament of language and of the profession, and in this way, suffices me in terms of ethical guidance.

Let me tell you about some of my experiences in that matter.

Following the Second World War, the establishment of an ethical framework was called upon as a necessity to help make sense of what had happened, and this was the impetus for the Declaration of Geneva, a kind of modern translation of the Hippocratic oath.

Doctors were in shock at the medical cruelty of the Holocaust, later referred to as the Shoah. The fascist eugenics policies instrumented in medicine from 1933 led to the euthanasia of many disabled individuals, to cruel and unspeakable scientific experiments on humans, and then to the Shoah.

Dr. Karl Brandt's law of protection of hereditary health was voted in 1933, six years prior to the war. The law permitted doctors to practice euthanasia for disabled children. At the same time, Dr. Asperger developed his ideas of social disabilities and autism in a psychiatric hospital in Vienna. During the Second World War, the hospital was transferring newly labelled "disabled" children to their death according to the law of protection of heredity health. Then, with the war and fascist roles, doctors like Josef Mengele used the pretext of science to commit atrocities on people in the concentration camps. Too many doctors took part in these atrocities. Some were condemned for crimes against humanity, while some escaped, like Josef Mengele.

After the war, the world looked back and tried to make sense of what happened, why and how. The leaders decided to create something that would ensure devilish law and systems could never happen again. They knew an international human law was necessary.

The United Nations was created and the Declaration of Geneva, a modern interpretation of the Hippocratic oath was pronounced.

The introduction 'With purity and with holiness I will pass my life and practice my art' was omitted from the declaration. Why? The law makers of the time probably wanted to clearly separate religion and morality. One could not rule the other in the modern world, I suppose. Furthermore, and most importantly, the creators of the United Nations needed to be universal, so that everyone, from Asia to Africa to the western world could accept and understand it. And in time, they did.

It was hoped that there would be no more Karl Brandts, Josef Mengeles or Dr. Aspergers, no more abuse of patients' rights and dignity in the name of science. Leaders of countries reacted too and set up social services and universal healthcare, to which we are now all accustomed. The French *Sécurité Sociale* was born in 1945 and the NHS in 1948. Doctors could embrace modern medicine, new technology and treatment through state-run universal care systems with the safety net of the Declaration of Geneva. 'Never again' was the motto of the time. Doctors were all optimistic and positivist. The profession could keep developing medical science with social justice and without the risk of unethical science.

The spirit of the time was helped by many new treatments and diagnostic tools. Chlorpromazine, the first tablet developed for psychiatric use, was discovered by Henry Laborit in 1952. Most antibiotics were also discovered between 1950 and 1970, and chlorothiazide, the first blood pressure treatment, appeared in 1958. At the same time, advances in medical knowledge, pre-op preparations, antiseptics and surgical care enabled surgeons to perform increasingly complex operations.

Then, about thirty years ago, one other metamorphosis happened. Medical care transformed itself with the adoption of a new ideology, called clinical evidence. Clinical evidence is based on results of studies and trials which are translated in guidelines for the physician to use. Since then, guidelines are again and again published with voracity for diagnosis, treatments, benefits and harms, and screening—actually, the whole medical field. Clinical evidence and its guidelines transformed the profession into a managerial techno-scientific process, focused on numbers, statistics and efficiency. With this change, the ethical rules got blurred again.

Dear Melo, I first heard about clinical evidence in 1999 in the UK. *Clinical evidence*, I thought. I've never heard of that before! When I understood what it was, I knew it would open the doors for so many more problems. As a medical student, I was taught never to forget that statistics were only an interpretation of the truth and not the truth itself. I was also taught that doctors needed to keep an independent view. They had to understand the limitations of statistics and identify the source of the results and potential bias. Clinical evidence is based on trials. The results of these treatments cannot stand as the whole story, as they only account for a fraction. It is a subjective and limited interpretation of statistical analysis from a third party. Subjectivity and conflict of interests cannot be ignored and, worse, cannot be understood by the physician. It is like doctors have lost access to and therefore the understanding of the truth behind the data.

That is what clinical evidence is, a pseudoscience, cutting the physician from the understanding of the data and perversely undermining the physician's trust in his or her own knowledge and experience. Sadly, a lot of my colleagues do not see these caveats. They just believe in clinical evidence as the one and only truth. Clinical evidence is an ideology. Sometimes I even get the impression that some of my colleagues are like religious believers. I cannot discuss the issue with them. I just cannot!

Now, let me tell you the two stories of today.

For my first placement as a student, I chose the general surgery at Antoine-Béclère Hospital. The hospital was in Clamart, on the southern outskirts of Paris, not far from Versailles. It was named after the founder of radiology in France back in 1895 and saw, in 1982, the birth of Amandine, the first ever French IVF baby. I do not know what happened in the hospital during the Second World War.

I was told that the culture of a hospital ward depended closely on the *chef de service*, head of the unit, and his or her personality. Professor Larrieu was considered an excellent surgeon with a big ego. He managed his unit with care and efficiency and was known to give an excellent grounding to his students. I felt privileged.

On that very first day, the professor welcomed us into a small room with bare walls, a tiny white desk and three chairs. The professor, the registrar by his side, faced us, the eight students. Everybody was standing quietly and respectfully. Doctors and students were all wearing the white coat, a symbol of cleanliness, natural authority and respect. Today, we do not wear it anymore. I must admit that I will always miss my white coat and often think of it with nostalgia.

The professor was tall, with grey hair, well-combed and parted on the side. His coat was immaculate. He had a stethoscope folded in his right pocket, a pen and a little black leather notebook in the left one. Underneath the coat, he had a cotton shirt and a dark tie. He was speaking such elegant French, I drank it in like others might drink Roger champagne. I swallowed his words and phrases. I wanted to remember them. I wanted to become him one day.

Professor Larrieu told us, 'The profession you have all chosen is a very difficult one indeed. It will be too challenging for some of you. During your studies and then your career, you will have numerous sleepless nights, not only because of the workload but also because of difficult or bad decisions you will have made or will have to make for someone else's life. However, if you treat each of your patients like one of your family members, not only will you be good doctors, but your life will be kinder, and you will sleep better.'

That was it. The professor had spoken. He just left us to our own thoughts and destinies.

All he gave us was this 'initiation lecture' to us doctors-to-be, and each of his words has remained in my brain to this day. This session was fundamental to my life and to my education. I had immediate trust in the profession I shall dedicate my life to.

I know, I know, this kind of lecture would today be considered too paternalistic and somewhat inappropriate. However, these simple words left a mark on my mind, forever.

Today, so many traditions and ways of respecting authority are out of fashion. That is what I call anomie. I have watched my profession changing radically. We have become so detached to those we care for. We don't treat people anymore; we treat medical conditions. As doctors, we now speak with acronyms and avoid any terminology linked to emotion. This is out of touch with medicine, you cannot just work with such language. The reality is that most of the time, doctors have to reassure people and, simultaneously, catch the fleeting moment to make decisions based on instinct and observation. We must interact with the person and our knowledge at the same time.

Some now refer to patients as subjects. The system is pushing us to see people as numbers and to classify human beings.

Dear Melo, I may be too negative; however, I often wonder what is good doctoring nowadays? Is the doctor of today equipped to reach decisions which are so important for the suffering human being in front of him or her?

And in reverse, does the doctor of today inspire trust?

Trust is not easily built between two human beings, let alone between a doctor and their patient. Sometimes, and I know this situation well, the patient will not trust the doctor at first sight. Then the wise words of Professor Larrieu cannot be of any help. And I realised this very early in my career.

Originally, I wanted to be a full specialist, to be an ophthalmologist, but to do so I would have had to return to school for another four years. Which I could not afford. So, I left Paris, and somewhat half-heartedly, went back to Brittany to do general medicine.

The practice I joined as a locum was in Huelgoat, a picturesque village in *les Monts d'Arrée*, the *Arrée* Mountains, surrounded by the remnants of the ancient Brittany Forest. The village was not far from Ploumilliau, my childhood village, only fifty-one kilometres away.

I got my first appointment in that village by pure chance. I was to replace a countryside doctor known for his skills in clinical diagnostics, just using his hands, mind and knowledge. His name was Dr. Gentile.

Let me tell you the story.

The day I met him he was wearing a suit but no tie. I was wearing a pencil skirt, high heels and a white shirt without the Hermes scarf I wore later in my career. At his first glance, I immediately understood and blushed: my high heels were frankly inappropriate. I reddened in silence and just sat down.

Dr. Gentile told me, 'Elpis, I remember my first locum work. I was exactly your age. It was on the island of Ouessant. I had to visit patients on horseback, you know. That sounds ancient and romantic, but it was difficult. The islanders were not easy, they were as harsh as the weather! However, the experience comforted me, to become a country doctor, far from the city and its stresses, close to real life, to rough humanity.'

I did not tell him that I myself was from the country, raised rough and on a farm. I felt awkward standing there like a proper Parisian, in my high heels.

Dr. Gentile then showed me around his practice and home in Huelgoat.

'Have you got any questions, Elpis?'

'Yes, Dr. Gentile.' I took a big breath and opened my heart about three matters that worried me most: time for diagnosis, driving and navigating at night, and dogs.

But Dr. Gentile told me, kindly, 'Fifteen minutes is more than enough. The trick is to control the patient's spoken words, to keep them to those most meaningful. And you should always take the opportunity to think in silence during the examination. That will allow time to build up your diagnosis. Always be confident and not over-stressed. I will tell you. A patient will never be offended if you say something like, 'I don't fully know what the problem is. Let me think about it and we'll review the situation tomorrow'.'

I thanked him and we carried on. I added, 'I am a bit concerned by home visits at night. So far, I have only driven in Paris. How would I find my way in the pitch-black night of the Arrée Mountains?'

The doctor replied with a calm, kind and comforting tone. With a smile on his face he said, 'You know, Elpis, country people are wiser than city dwellers. You can rely on them. The farmers will always light their home to direct you, the doctor.'

'Thank you. And what about dogs?'

'Do not worry. Dangerous dogs are locked up, especially when a doctor is expected. If the animal is left outside, it is not a dangerous one. Simple, no?'

I listened respectfully and carefully. Then, I was shown the home I was to stay in for the next two weeks.

Dr. Gentile's surgery was an extension of his home. The plan was that I would eat and sleep there. The surgery itself was a suite of three rooms. The waiting room was on the north side, connected to the doctor's office by a dark corridor of about 10 metres. The examination room was linked to the doctor's office by a door. There were two exits to the outside, one from the waiting room and one from the doctor's office. Patients leaving the doctor did not see the patients still awaiting their turn. Clever design, I thought.

I joined Dr. Gentile and his family for dinner. They were supposed to leave the next day for their ski holiday. After an animated and welcoming family dinner, everyone retired to their bedrooms early. I went to bed with my Dorosz to read about antibiotics. I did not fall asleep easily. I tossed and turned, feeling both anxious and excited.

Then the first day of my general practice began.

I was feeling stressed and out of balance after a sleepless night. But here I was, at the doctor's desk, one hour before my consultation. I double-checked I had everything I needed: several pens, my stethoscope, one medical light, a sphygmomanometer, tongue depressors and one otoscope.

I had a batch of fifty forms to fill in, and cash to give change. As opposed to my work at the hospital, each consultation would have to be concluded by a payment which should be exchanged against a form the patient would then send to the *Sécurité Sociale* to be reimbursed.

This was the ritual I had to get used to.

On the left side of the desk, I carefully laid down my precious Dorosz, the medication thesaurus and my holy grail. French medical students used to call it 'the red book', I called it my holy grail, though secretly. It was bigger than Mao's red book, yet small enough to fit in the pocket of a doctor's white coat.

But I was not wearing a white coat. The pocket for my Dorosz was not available. I paused and opted for a place on the desk and respectfully put my precious companion there on the left.

9 am. Time for the first patient. I walked down the faintly lit corridor to the waiting room in seven quick, bold steps, and then opened the door with a determined movement. Melo, the waiting room was full of people sitting and several standing. There were about thirty people waiting for the doctor, but not for me, Elpis, a young girl doctor with high heels, *une debutante*!

I managed to remain calm though, murmured a '*Bonjour Messieurs, Dames,*' then invited the first patient to follow me to the consulting room.

I have forgotten the diagnosis I made. I just recall looking after the man the same way I had done at the hospital.

Then I showed him the exit before I literally ran back the other way to the corridor. I went to open the door of the waiting room, ready to invite the next patient in. I felt triumphant. I was thinking that I would see all these people, one by one, this very morning. I would do it; I could do it!

Impossible, incredible! *Incroyable!* No one was there!

To my astonishment, everyone had gone! They had all left! The sick villagers just did not trust me, the young Parisian girl with high heels."

Melo stopped writing, raised her gaze, and murmured, "Doctor, really, did they all leave?"

"Yes, Melo, they all escaped. I must admit that at the age of twenty-four I looked only sixteen! I did not look like a doctor at all. I was petite, with a cherub's face, and inquisitive round eyes. The high heels did not help either! Not a country doctor's look, really. I can understand my physiognomy did not inspire confidence at first sight, let alone trust. But I was so upset, so shocked.

Years later, I cannot remember what I did for the rest of the morning. Dear Melo, I have never told anyone that. It was a secret, one I am now sharing with you.

I understand that first impressions matter when you go to see a doctor for the first time. I discovered this lesson that day. I knew that I had to appear more mature and professional. No more high heels.

While I was buried in my solitude and despair in my new, patient-less office, the secretary came to me. She gave me a list of home visits and showed me two pairs of shoes Dr. Gentile had asked her to bring. One pair suited me; they were a pair of black, Clarke shoes. I thanked her but did not tell the woman that I had seen only one patient, that the others had escaped from me! I suppose I was too upset and proud to do so.

However, I stayed in Huelgoat and soon saw other patients.

Melo, appearance in work is important. It must suit your practice and what you do. Whether we like it or not, we must look a certain way to gain the trust of others. Trust requires sacrifice, and trusting yourself requires risk. But we'll get to that next week."

The meeting had ended as it always did, and as Dr. Elpis stood from the table and left The Mirage, Melo left soon after. She took her cherry-red bike and cycled a shorter path home. She was eager to go back home and talk to her father. Then, she remembered he was gone, away for the next week or so.

Melo wanted to reflect on today's meeting before writing. She was interested in how people gave trust to Hippocrates and Asclepius, compared to what Dr. Elpis had told her that day. She perceived the potential dangers of mixing religious beliefs with medicine. She felt the need to read and thought of Dr. Hart's illustrated book in the library. Melo wanted to learn.

When Melo arrived at home, she left her bike in the garage and walked up the stairs to the kitchen. It was closed. Her mother was not at home. She left the garage, walked through the garden to the main entrance and opened the door with her own key, the one she always kept attached to a chain on her backpack.

Her mother left a note on the kitchen table: 'I shall be late today, I am meeting Anna and her husband in Chelsea, do not wait for me, there is plenty of food in the fridge, love you.'

She read the note and thought, *typical*. She will not call her mother. Rather, she decided to go and get the book from the library. She was sure her father would not mind.

Melo left her glass half-full near her mother's note and walked through the corridor to the library. She opened the door, and did not make any noise, as if her father's spirit was still in the room. She did not want to disturb anything or anyone connected to that space. That was a must.

She closed the door with the same quietness and walked upon the Persian rug with its tree of life, moving her feet with lightness and delicacy. The space was dark, except for a couple rays of light sneaking through the persiennes. Melo went directly to the mahogany cocktail table where the book was last, felt the need to face the *Hakushiko* mask but did not dare.

To her surprise, the book was not there. Melo froze, stopped like at a loss. She felt she had been tricked. The book should have been on that table. She did not know where to go; she did not want to sneak around her father's office. She did not want to intrude on his intimate place any more than she already had. She turned back towards the exit with the same light feet, and as her head turned, she caught the book in her visual periphery. It was on her father's desk, just in front of his chair. Melo went and grabbed the book, left the room quickly and quietly closed the door behind her. The pressure went. She left no trace of her intrusion behind.

Melo walked up the stairs to her room and took a seat at her desk. She opened the book and quickly found what she was looking for. She flipped to page ninety-one, the chapter about votives, the offerings ancient Greeks used to give to the temples in recognition of Asclepius' good treatment. She began to read about the ancient connection between medical care, trust and holiness. This was her way to connect with the depth of Dr. Elpis' stories.

I will follow that system of regimen which,
according to my ability and judgment, I consider
for the benefit of my patients, and abstain from
whatever is deleterious and mischievous

HIPPOCRATES

Saturday Six

On the seventh Saturday, Melo the anthropologist felt somewhat closer to medicine, a noble profession indeed. She now knew that the Hippocratic oath meant much more than 'do no harm'. Her father was correct: people oversimplified the oath. Its original message got lost in translation. Despite the fact that it's dated, it was clear to Melo—as it always had been to Elpis—that the message was valid, eternal and universal. Although complex in its nature, it perfectly surrounded medical ethics, just like an origin myth.

The anthropologist was also interested to know that the most recent revival of the oath, named the Declaration of Geneva, happened not long ago, in 1948, following the Second World War, the holocaust and Dr. Asperger's discovery of autism. Melo had first heard the word Asperger at the time of her diagnosis at the age of eight. She was brought in for a consultation because of the way she was not socialising at school. As a matter of fact, Melo acted that way *not* because of her inner life, but because the girls that surrounded her at that time talked and talked like parrots, rudely and repetitively. Her father understood this. He felt that psychologists were out of order in education. As soon as he heard them speaking about Melo as if she had a disability, he knew they were wrong. This was just a narrative they pushed because they could not understand it. Melo's father felt that it was a gift to not be normal for psychologists, he knew the gift that Melo was.

Melo's father was comforted by his beliefs when he read that Lorna Wing regretted introducing the label 'Asperger's' for the less intense side of the disability. Lorna Wing was an eminent, intelligent psychologist and a mother of a daughter with severe autism, so much so that her little girl could not speak. Wing wanted to demonstrate that there were different intensities of the diagnosis, and that kids with apparently normal speaking and learning capabilities could have a form of autism too. So, she introduced the notion of spectrum. What she wanted to do was attract a lot of attention and wanted schools and doctors to be able to identify possible autism. This led to a damaging overdiagnosis of autism and the abuse of that diagnosis in education.

She believed she had found a solution, that all she had done was well-intentioned. But buried underneath all of this was an idea of disability. Lorna Wing expanded the notion of 'the other,' the same notion that made Melo's father pull her from school as a child. Melo may have Asperger's, but she did not have a disability. Without her father, she may have fallen victim to the idea that she did. It was the labelling that was wrong. It was the labelling that made people 'other.'

When Lorna Wing retired, she wrote an article documenting her regret for expanding the spectrum of autism and using the name Asperger for two reasons. Firstly, when her beliefs were accepted into society, schools made a change. Now that the spectrum was so wide, many kids were placed onto it. There was an inflation of diagnosis, and suddenly a huge amount of kids were being labelled and some-times separated from their peers on the basis that they were 'disabled.' A whole generation of children were affected negatively because of this. Lorna said she had opened a Pandora's Box. This escalated when Dr. Asperger's role in the euthanasia of disabled children was revealed to the world over fifty years after the fact. This truth furthered the negative effect of Lorna Wing's initial good intentions.

Melo pondered all of this as she prepared for the seventh Saturday with Dr. Elpis. With that same unshaken, confident spirit, she went. Melo did not take her cherry-red bike because she had to collect a laudanum silk dress for her mother at A Child of the Jago in Covent Garden, not far from The Mirage, after the meeting that day. Apparently, and according to her mother, the UK brand was inspired by A Child of the Jago's heroes and was a response to fight fast fashion. She decided to venture once again through the underground.

After she resurfaced from the escalators, she began her usual route.

She was smiling, head in the clouds, as she walked up Carnaby Street, passing by Rags and Bones, turning on Greek Street and heading down Bateman Crook Lane. The Mirage was in the distance.

Mia was setting up the tables outside when Melo arrived. The sky was already clear blue, with just a few scattered altostratus clouds above.

"Good morning, Melo."

"Mia, do you know the Crocobar?"

"What?"

"The Crocobar, the bar with metal music?"

"Ah yes, it's a bit dodgy though."

"A few of my bandmates have been talking about it, but I've never been. Would you want to go with me some night?"

The young waitress gazed at Melo and raised her small perky nose and replied in a very matter of fact way, "Melo! I can't believe it, are you actually asking to go out and be seen in the world? With me? I'd love to go, we can discuss next week. The doctor is waiting for you, I'll bring your tea."

The two girls entered as one, Melo headed to the back while Mia went behind the bar.

The doctor began.

"Good morning, do take a seat. No bike today?"

"No, I have to go shopping after our meeting. Do you know A Child of the Jago? The main store is just around the corner from here."

"A Child of the Jago? I have never heard of it."

A few minutes of silence settled. Then, Melo said,

"Dr. Elpis, I look forward to the next story in Huelgoat. Poor you, that must have been hard, to work with those farmers after such a terrible first day. I tried to imagine how the waiting room emptied. Did one person leave first and then another one? Or did they all conspire and decide to leave at once?"

"We will never know, Melo. Yes, it was a huge blow indeed. But I was young, intrepid and fearless. I was already proud and strong, you know.

And the story I am about to tell tested my strength just as much."

Melo pulled the Moleskine notebook and the pen box out of her bag. She took out one of the pens with care and gazed at the doctor with wide-open green eyes. Elpis was so tiny, as if she was barely alive under the hood. She was immobile, both hands still on the table, palms down. Melo stared at the hooded face and imaginary *Hakushiko* mask with its peaceful smile.

With her beautiful and very peaceful voice, the doctor started,

"So, after the first terrible affront to my vanity, the Huelgoat people began to consult with me. They did not have any other option! As Dr. Gentile's replacement, I was the only doctor who could care for them. Fortunately, the few patients I saw got some benefits from my care. I treated them well. People gossiped though, as they always do. It was said, that Dr.Gentile was better, and that anyway he was coming back soon.

It was the evening of the seventh day. I had to visit a widower. I was told he was living alone and was not well. He needed to see the doctor.

7 pm. I drove my white three-door hatchback Mk2 Ford Fiesta in the pitch-black night. A few minutes after having left the village, I followed the single light up a hill. This must be the widower's home, I thought. And so, I drove towards the light in the pitch-dark countryside.

As I arrived, I parked the car alongside the wall, on the limits of the property. When I opened the door, I heard barking. As I turned my head towards the light and the house, a ginormous, scary German shepherd stood waiting for me in the dark. I felt his presence as soon as my foot hit the ground. I knew he was waiting for me.

I played Dr. Gentile's wise words in my mind and focused on them. 'If a dog is left outside, it is not a dangerous one.' But when the dog charged at me and was at my feet, I found it difficult to feel calm as the animal sniffed me out.

I knew I could not afford another affront. I could not. I knew the way the people of the town saw me already, and I did not want them to think I feared a dog, even a huge barking black one. Besides, a sick man was waiting for me.

So, I stood my ground and walked resolutely towards the lit farm door, the vicious-looking canine by my side continuing to sniff and bark intermittently. I tried not to look into the animal's eyes, but when he flashed his teeth and let out another awful bark—truthfully—I was scared.

I tried to forget about my feelings. At the same time, I was careful to not mess up my French lookalike Wellington boots in the muddy path. A little voice in my head said, '*Elpis, hang on, you are a doctor. Do not get dismissed for any reason, not again, be strong!*'

I was determined and, despite the fear, I felt courageous. The dog would not attack me, would not bite or eat me, and I would do my work as I should! Darkness and dogs would not deter me; I would follow the light.

After this infinitely long walk across the courtyard, the dog and I were at the door of the widower's home. Before I had the opportunity to knock, a giant, grey-haired old man opened the door, and with one head movement invited me in. As I entered, the dog was left behind. Now, I could do my job. The man's face was craggy, stern and sad, with quiet blue eyes. I immediately began taking note of him and his movements. He was limping.

I sat on the bench at the rectangular wood table, with its red and yellow multiflora oil cloth. The fire was roaring in the large open fireplace, with at least two days' worth of cut birch wood at the side. The place was well kept. I could smell a leek and potato soup. The table was cleared of food, except for the rectangular biscuit tin with blue and yellow folkloric dancers. This was the traditional Briton farmer's safe, always positioned carefully at the centre when the doctor arrived. The giant went to his chair and waited for me.

He was wearing soft, navy-blue cotton trousers, a cedar and cinnamon check shirt, and a cable-knit, gingerbread-brown cardigan. I turned to face the man. Without a word, he pulled up his trouser leg, revealing a shiny, swelled-up lower limb.

'It aches,' he said. 'It just swelled up yesterday for no reason. I've stayed at home since I left the hospital last week. My daughter comes every day for the food and the animals. I don't understand it.'

I looked at him and observed. His left arm was weak. The faint limping and slow movements I'd first noticed came back to my mind. After a few seconds of observation, I asked,

'Why were you at the hospital?'

'I had a stroke, they said. But I am alright now, my left hand's a bit weak, that's all.'

I got closer, put both hands skilfully around the swelled-up, shiny, red leg and spread my fingers to feel the consistency and hardness just below the skin. It was more hard than soft from the ankle to the middle of the calf.

I kept silent, touching and thinking. In the absence of injury, the three possible diagnoses were: One, a deep venous thrombosis. Two, a cardiac, liver or kidney failure. Three, a skin infection called cellulitis.

I kept silent and thought while I checked the other leg. No oedema, no redness. I then took my stethoscope and sphygmomanometer and checked his blood pressure, then listened to his heart. I inserted a mercury thermometer into the man's mouth. The temperature was 36.5 degrees Celsius; he didn't have a fever. I could not examine the abdomen in this position, but thanks to my hospital training, I felt confident enough to know for sure that Pierre did not have any ascites (swelling of the abdomen). He did not have swelling on the other leg either. His blood pressure and heart were both Ok. I concluded that it could not be a heart, kidney, or liver issue. I then asked him to take off his slipper and sock. A clean, immaculate foot was shown with no sign of athlete's foot or other damage. Cellulitis was unlikely with that foot, especially in the absence of a fever.

Of course, I got it. This was a deep venous thrombosis. Pierre had been in a hospital bed for two weeks. In that time, a stroke was not treated as it is nowadays. There was no immediate cure, scans were not done routinely. The doctor, along with the patient, just had to hope that the damage would be limited, and that time would heal.

I was happy to have made such a good diagnosis away from the hospital and on my own. I looked the giant right in his eyes and announced, with triumph,

'I am afraid you have a deep venous thrombosis. You have to go back to the hospital for treatment.'

I remember. Pierre gazed back at me, right into my eyes, and bluntly replied, 'I am not going back to the hospital, not ever again.'

I did not lower my gaze, but I was at a loss. I could not consult with a fellow family member or friend. There was no one else I could talk to. I took a deep breath, lowered my gaze towards the swelling red shiny thrombosis, and finally replied, 'Let me think about it, I'll come tomorrow, early afternoon.'

The giant then put his sock and slipper back on and lowered his trouser over his leg. Meanwhile, I went to clean my hands. Back at the table, I sat down and took a social security form from my doctor's bag. Respectfully, and with subtle care, Pierre opened the metallic biscuit tin and took out twenty francs to pay for my consultation. I filled in the form and receipt for payment. With deference, Pierre took the form for reimbursement in exchange for the twenty francs. I put the note in my leather wallet.

I stood, put my precious stethoscope and sphygmomanometer in the black leather medical bag, put my coat on and, in silence, I left Pierre. I knew the dog would be waiting so I crossed the yard quickly, trying to beat the dog to my car. I nearly slipped in the mud as we raced. Once I made it to the car, I jumped in, slammed the door, and took a deep breath of relief. I could not hear the dog barking anymore.

Once I arrived home, I went straight to my room and called Dr. Gentile at once. It was 8 pm, but I guessed he would not be offended to be called for advice, even during his holiday.

'*Bonsoir Docteur, c'est Elpis. Voila, j'ai un problème.* I went to see Pierre. He left the hospital last week, Dr. Gentile, I am certain he has a deep venous thrombosis. He needs to go back to the hospital, but he does not want to. I'm worried about giving him heparin or even the new treatment, its low weight molecular counterpart. It is written in the Dorosz and also in the Vidal in your office: if the stroke was a bleeding one, he could die. If it wasn't, the treatment will save him.'

Dr. Gentile replied, 'You are not going to let him die from his thrombosis, are you? I do not think you have many options, I'm afraid.'

'Thank you, Doctor, for taking the call. I understand. I will go back to see him tomorrow and will do my job, you can count on me.'

I put down the phone, at a bit of a loss. I recomposed myself and got ready for supper. I tried to relax in front of the television but did not stay long. I was too exhausted. Instead, I retired to the bedroom. It was freezing cold, so I stripped down to my naked self and snaked under the red taffeta eiderdown and my yellow blanket. The linen was fresh, washed only yesterday. My body felt good and warmed up instantly. In a few seconds, I was sleeping and dreaming.

The next day, I drove back to the farm. The place was different in the daylight. The path from the parking to the main building was 50 metres long, no more. The mud had dried up, making the walk a lot easier. A few hens were pecking in freedom, and swine could be heard grunting and squealing.

The dog was different in the daylight. He looked smaller, and less frightening. His white teeth didn't stick out in the darkness. I could see him and he could see me. He remembered my scent from the night before. It was like he knew I was the doctor and that I would care for his master.

Once again, Pierre opened the door before I had to knock.

I examined the man and prescribed the low weight molecular heparin, a brand-new treatment at the time. I did the first injection and said that the nurse would have to come every day for the next few weeks and repeat the injection. He agreed.

'I will come back to see you in five days.'

Then I left and crossed the courtyard, the dog by my side.

I must admit, I did not sleep well the following four nights. I was tossing and turning. The fresh-smelling linen did not have the same hypnotic effect from the previous night. My mind could not rest. Pierre had had a stroke, but was it a bleeding one? If so, my treatment, away from the hospital, would soon be detrimental. It would aggravate the bleeding and the stroke. My treatment could kill the man, nothing less. I could not know. I could only guess and hope. Only what came next would tell. And it did.

Monsieur Pierre hadn't had a bleeding stroke, just an ischaemic one. He recovered from both thrombosis and stroke, thanks to the treatment I prescribed.

Dear Melo, one Hippocratic aphorism is as follows:

Life is short, science is long; opportunity is elusive, experiment is dangerous, judgement is difficult. It is not enough for the physician to do what is necessary, but the patient and the attendants must do their part as well, and circumstances must be favourable.

Twenty-five centuries later, I could not agree more. Hippocrates had many of these aphorisms which help us to understand beyond 'Do No Harm.' Non-maleficence can be difficult to define sometimes. In the case of Pierre, it was not right for me to prescribe this medicine at home, but what I did was correct. I could not force the man from his home and into the hospital. I had to push the boundaries. That is the real world!

And, according to the Hippocratic oath, *I will follow that system of <u>regimen</u> which, according to my ability and judgment, I consider for the benefit of my patients, and abstain from whatever is <u>deleterious</u> and mischievous.*

I treated Pierre: widower, farmer, father and dog owner according to my ability and judgment. I evaluated all the components of the situation and opted to treat the man in respect of his wishes and dignity.

The most important part of this story is that Pierre recovered. My treatment allowed him to live out a healthy life, and I did not force him to do anything against his will. It was a mutual respect of one another. I had to trust myself, and then he learned to trust me. This is what I repeat in my profession, over and over. This likely contributed to the change in tone of the gossip of the town from the high-heeled girl to an honourable doctor."

Melo nodded in acknowledgment of the end of the story. She said goodbye to the doctor, and the doctor said goodbye to her. Elpis left, while Melo walked down to the bar where Mia was setting new bottles on shelves.

With resolution and courage, Melo stopped and faced the bar.

"Mia, if I bring my bike next week, will you help me again?"

"Sure, Melo, see you on Saturday." Mia winked at the blogger and got back to sorting out the shelves.

Melo left, a smile on her face, curls bouncing while catching sun rays as she left The Mirage.

▲

On the Monday before the next meeting, Melo went to the cinema with her mother to see Quentin Tarantino's latest movie *Once Upon a Time in Hollywood*. The whole family has been a fan of Quentin since Jackie Brown's film, so much so that Melo saw the whole Kill Bill trilogy at the age of eight.

She woke up late the following day since there was no early meeting to attend. She went downstairs to have breakfast with her laptop in hand. Her mother was sipping a cup of tea, reading The Telegraph. Her father still hadn't returned from Japan but was due back this weekend.

"Good morning my dolly, did you sleep well? I enjoyed the film last night. I have not made up my mind on the ending though. I find Tarantino a bit cynical, with the whole violent, psycho cult slash hippie counterculture of the sixties."

Melo replied while pouring the milk on her cornflakes.

"They were all druggy, Mom."

Her mother did not reply, just sighed, putting her glasses back on to read. Melo started to eat while checking her morning emails.

One was from the doctor. Unusual. Elpis asked Melo to change the rendezvous location and time to the New Forest this coming Saturday morning at 10 am. The doctor informed her she would have a driver pick her up from the Weymouth train station. Melo was unsure if this would be possible, as her father's return from Japan was planned on that very day at 6 pm at the Heathrow airport. Would it be possible for Melo to do both? Be in the New Forest in the morning and then go to welcome her father at night?

Mother and daughter discussed the issue and made a plan. Melo will go to the New Forest by train for the meeting at 10 am, meet her mother at 12.30 am for a pub lunch to then drive to Heathrow airport from the country. That will work, they both agreed. Her mother was happy to go to the New Forest anyway. It was an opportunity to drive her brand-new hybrid car and to wear her new dress from A Child of the Jago.

Melo sent an email of reply to the doctor. The time and location were both agreeable. She was looking forward to being somewhere new. She sent a text to her father with the change of plan for his arrival date. He replied with a big red heart and a grey doctor examining it with his stethoscope. She smiled at the emoji. She was amazed and positive about her father's recent interest in the digital symbols. It was that interest that brought him to the conference in Japan. Even as a linguist trained in ancient languages, her father understood the impact of emojis in digital communication. Emojis transcend both language barriers and technology limits. They enhance modern communication prompting cultural hybridisation. For Melo, this was obvious. With emojis, a silent text becomes organic, colourful and joyful, and instant emotional connection just happens between two people so far away from each other, like Melo and her father, she, in London, and he, in Tokyo. After receiving the emoji on her iPhone, Melo googled the distance as the crow flies between London and Tokyo. It was exactly 9566 kilometres. The young woman was amazed. So far, and yet, immediate emotional communication.

Melo was happy discovering and enthralled with her anthropologist work around medicine. She spent the rest of the week reading the oath and Dr. Hart's Book, *Asclepius: The God of Medicine*. She kept the book in her bedroom, just close to the Hippocratic oath.

I will not cut persons laboring under the stone, but will leave this to be done by men who are practitioners of this work.

HIPPOCRATES

Saturday Seven

At 9.27 on Saturday morning, Melo arrived at Weymouth station in the New Forest. A tall, blond man was already waiting for her. She followed him to a lookalike Cadillac door as he welcomed her to the country. Inside the car, the windows were tinted. This, as the driver explained, was to ensure the anonymity of the doctor's whereabouts. The estate had to remain a secret.

The driver reminded Melo of Cliff Booth from *Once Upon a time in Hollywood*. He was a quiet man with a Cadillac car, just like Cliff. She wondered if he was a friendly dog lover too. They rode for about twenty minutes until coming upon a gate that opened as they drove in. The car stopped, and the driver came to the back to open the door for Melo. When she stepped foot on the ground, she looked around to see a perfectly maintained garden with several ancient oaks and an alley of olive trees forming a path to a terrace opposite to a grazing field for horses. Olive trees together with ancient oaks in the British New Forest, Melo thought. Her mother was correct. Climate was changing in a big way! That was real, whatever the reasons.

While walking, Melo also thought of Mia. She regretted not telling her that she would not be at The Mirage today. She missed her. Melo felt close to Mia; a real friendship was developing, nothing virtual but something real. She'd never had a friend before and had never been close to someone other than her family members. Having been home-schooled, she never had the chance to really meet people until her university time in Durham. But even at university, she'd managed to keep to herself and limit social contact to the minimum. Melo was happy with her life though. She enjoyed being in crowds when she got to be the observer. This was the reason why she chose to be an anthropologist, rather than a journalist. Mia was the first person to ever single her out in a friendly way and make Melo feel like she could have a one-to-one connection. And this was becoming apparent to her as she felt Mia's absence here in the New Forest. She was missing her friend.

Melo reached the end of the pathway and turned to the side of the house to see Dr. Elpis on the terrace sitting at a table. It was blue skies above, two horses were 10 metres away, approaching the fence to face the doctor.

"Dear Melo, good morning, so nice to see you."

Without any small talk, Melo set up her notebook and chose one of her three pens from the box. The doctor started.

"Serendipity has been in action this week. The patient I am about to tell the story of came to see me just three days ago. I had to explain our work, I had to. I had to be sure he knows we were respecting his privacy. The man is called Kevin. He welcomed the idea with emotion. He even shed a tear and, out of the blue, sang the Irish song *This Story I Tell You Is True* right there in my office.

He told me I had saved his life and was delighted that I was telling the story. However, the man was not saved by me alone, no, he was saved by humanist medicine in all its glory. Each professional involved in his care did what they were trained to do at the right time and in accordance with each other's actions. All limited their parts to their own competence and cooperated according to the Hippocratic oath's words, *I will not cut persons laboring under the stone, but will leave this to be done by men who are practitioners of this work.*"

Dr. Elpis moved slightly into a more comfortable seated position, then said, "Melo, before I start, I must first point out the complexity of medical care today. One can count at least eighty specialities, surgical or medical, with even more subspecialties. Doctors work in connection with other professions too, from podiatrists to psychologists, social workers to technicians of all sorts. Most of the time, one case is dealt with by various experts at the same time. For example, it is not unusual to have one surgeon working with one anaesthetist, two radiologist consultants, technicians, nurses, and even a robot in one surgical theatre around one single patient. Today, one hopes that patients do not get lost in between and that mistakes are prevented by cooperation between each specialist, who must appropriately know their limits according to the ancient wisdom. In Harley Street, healthcare is dealing with anything from cosmetic surgery to complex surgery and advance medical treatment.

So.

One morning, I was preparing to go to my office on Harley Street and took my usual route from the gym. I crossed Golden Square, then went on to Carnaby Street to stop for some morning porridge with a little pot of honey, a small ham sandwich and a green tea from the local Pret a Manger. It was my special day of the week with breakfast out. I sat outside and watched the life passing by. The day was starting in Carnaby Street.

A tall woman with long, pink hair and a backpack was walking down the street. A man with a suit and wireless earphones in his ears was passing by talking to the empty space around him. Two mates with long hair walked along the other side of the street. A homeless man, his hair all messed up, his eyes barely open, looking for a coin or two to get his morning coffee. A man and a woman in smart working clothes walked together, each of them with a laptop bag in hand, like clones of one another.

Savouring the buzz and the diversity of it all, I ate everything in twenty minutes. I had to leave.

With my Asics on, I walked briskly along Liberty to Regent Street toward Oxford Circus. A few minutes later, I was on Cavendish Square. Harley Street was on the horizon with two straight lines of buildings four to five floors high ahead. There were altocumulus clouds in the sky above. A plane was crossing overhead. The roads were busy. I crossed Cavendish Square, then Wigmore Street, only a few yards away from my office building. As I arrived closer, the scaffolding began blocking the view.

Harley Street was busy. Food was being delivered. Cars were being parked. I saw my friend and colleague parking his black Moto Guzzi.

Pedestrians and patients were many. Husband and wife were pushing their tiny, sick child in a wheelchair, and a frail lady with a desperate Hippocratic face was being helped up the stairs of the next building. Two women wearing fashion from tip to toe and makeup for Instagram were getting out of an Uber car. That was the diversity in Harley Street.

I spotted one other colleague from across the street parking his Malbec red metallic Touareg Volkswagen. Another friend, a dermatologist consultant, wearing his usual exquisite bowtie, waved hello to me from across the street.

'Good morning, Elpis.'

'Good morning *mon ami*.'

Harley Street's start of the weekday, I suppose.

I arrived at my office at 9.55 am. I took off my coat and changed my shoes for my MaxMara high-heeled sandals. I got to my desk and logged on to my computer. The files for the day were already to my left. The morning was fully booked until 1 pm.

I went through my routine and saw about five people that morning. When I was about to take my lunch break, my assistant informed me that Kevin had just shown up for help. He was a patient of mine that I had taken care of for nearly twenty years. I could not refuse to see him. I asked the receptionist to send him in. My tummy was already rumbling, but I knew I had to see Kevin. I had to be ready and available for the unexpected.

Kevin, the tall man with Celtic genes, sat down and said, 'Dr. Elpis, I was cycling and felt a sharp pain there in my...'

As these words were said, the man pointed at his skull and then just ... collapsed. His head banged on my desk. I froze. Then a seizure agitated the unconscious man for two to three seconds. I understood immediately what was happening: an excessive, hyper synchronous discharge of neurons occurred as the result of an insult to the brain. The man took a big breath with a deep worrying noise. Was he gasping? When someone unconscious begins to breathe irregularly with this sound, it is a sign of imminent death.

In a second, I jumped from my desk and reached the man on the floor. Instinctively, I shouted, 'Kevin, can you hear me?' The man began seizing again, and then vomited. I knew he was having a subarachnoid haemorrhage, in other words, a brain haemorrhage. I knew what was happening.

I visualised the blood invading the brain's cavities and ventricles, effectively drowning the brain. At that moment, the brain must have already begun reacting by producing excessive electrical discharges in the enclosed skull, hence the convulsions.

In one learned movement, I pushed Kevin onto his side and opened his airway by tilting his head and lifting the chin. I checked his breathing and felt for his pulse on his neck. He was breathing, his pulse was palpable. There was no need for cardiopulmonary resuscitation. No need for a defibrillator either.

I yelled, 'Help, help!'

My assistant appeared. I told him to keep checking the pulse and breathing exactly as he has been trained to do. As he kneeled down on the side of Kevin's body in one movement, I went to the other side of my desk and picked up the phone to dial 999.

'I am at 2000 Harley Street, postcode HIP0 5BC. I am Dr. Elpis and a man of sixty-five has collapsed in my office. His pulse is detectable and regular.'

'Is he breathing?'

'Yes.'

'Can you count the breathing for me now, please.'

'One, two … three. I believe he has a subarachnoid haemorrhage.'

'Stay with the patient, we are coming.'

Four minutes later, the sound of the ambulance's siren broke Harley Street's familiar background noise. The paramedic squad entered the building, equipped with all the necessary resuscitation materials and a stretcher. The skilled people questioned me while assessing the unconscious man and setting up an IV access. Meanwhile, in one movement, I was back at my computer on the other side of the desk, writing a report for the hospital. My receptionist kept the corridor free from other people, politely pushed away curious eyes and talked to Kevin's driver who was now in. In seven minutes, the patient was put on the stretcher, his body connected to an ECG and BP monitor. The infusion was set in his arm. He was ready for the ambulance transfer to the hospital. The receptionist, my assistant and I surrounded to help and balance the stretcher along the corridor, through the door and down the stairs outside. In a concerted move-ment, we held off the stretcher and left it to the paramedics and the ambulance. We stood speechless and transfixed as we watched the departing ambulance drive Kevin away. Then in silence, we walked back to work.

I went to my office and sat down at the desk with all the chaos left after the major event, the near-death of my patient, nothing less. I remembered to stay there for a few minutes and then left for lunch without a word. Once at home, I did not eat much though.

The family was informed. Kevin had suffered a grade 5 brain haemorrhage.

The scanner showed what I had envisioned earlier: a brain's hae-morrhage with a hydrocephalus. Blood was filling the subarachnoid spaces, the closed spaces surrounded by the brain. The culprit, a burst aneurysm—the initial cause of the event—was visualised on the CT scan. The aneurysm was a genetic localised abnormality, a weak spot on the wall and the lining of the artery. And on that day, out of the blue, the aneurysm had burst.

The man would probably not get through this. The prognosis was bad.

However, he was operated on. With the purpose of resolving the hydrocephalus—and to release the pressure on the brain—a left frontal, extra ventricular drain was inserted by the highly skilled neurosurgeon alongside his team of anaesthetists, technicians and nurses. The next day, a coil embolization of the actual burst aneurysm was performed to seal it for good. The surgeon skilfully inserted a hollow plastic tube called a catheter into an artery in the groin to thread it through the body, to reach Kevin's aneurysm at the base of the brain. Thereafter, he used the catheter to push a soft platinum wire into the aneurysm. The wire coiled up inside the aneurysm, disrupted the blood flow and sealed off the bulging from the artery, hopefully for good. Finally, and as an extra precaution, a right-sided, ventriculoperitoneal shunt was inserted. This was to ensure immediate release of pressure in the eventuality of further bleeding.

Amazingly and wonderfully, Kevin survived.

He had some complications though, with right-sided chest effusion, swallowing difficulties and an impaired memory. He stayed in the neurosurgery ward for three months. Kevin was never left alone. Every day, his wife and other family members would be by his side.

And each time I went to see him I thought of them all as a heroic family of the twenty-first century.

In time, all complications were resolved by good care and technology. Kevin got transferred to the rehabilitation centre, where he stayed for a further three months. Amazingly, the man recovered his physical and mental autonomy. A limited amnesia remained though. Everything that happened from November had been erased from his memory forever. What happened to him at my office will never be part of his past in his mind. That is why, Melo, we should both be honoured to know and write down his story.

In the end, Kevin chose not to return to running his flourishing business. He took his medication regularly and saw the doctors according to plan.

He now lives mostly in Kerry County of Ireland, his home, with his trusted wife and my humble advice 'Do work on your farm. Enjoy your family life. Connect with nature, enjoy. You deserve it.'

The year following Kevin's rescue, I went to his son's wedding celebration at Killarney. I was delighted to have been invited and looked forward to seeing the family reunited in their home far from London, the hospital and Harley Street.

Before the plane from London landed, I looked through the window and recognised the mountain range called the Macgillycuddy's Reeks and the River Shannon. The Celtic coastline was rough from the sky, just like the Brittany coast I know so well. I could not figure out where the famous Skellig Islands were though. I read a lot about the monks who built beehive-shaped, stone huts clinging on the cliffs centuries ago. I could not see the Islands from the plane and was a bit lost with my history too. I wondered if these religious people were contemporary to the monks and eremites who braved the sea and emigrated from Ireland to Brittany to bring Christianity to my pagan ancestors. I did not know. But I wondered.

I arrived safely at my hotel and got prepared for the festivities.

On the first day of celebrations, we all gathered for dinner. Following much food and drink, a few important, emotional words were spoken.

'My special son … his beautiful, special chosen one … our parents and grandparents … our friends … when he was a boy … when she was a girl …' The usual things people talk about on a wedding day, all around the world.

Next, a young boy, Kevin's grandson of twelve, stood up to speak.

With solemnity and dignity, the young boy in a perfectly fitted suit and tie, addressed all with power and clarity.

'I want to thank Dr. Elpis for saving the life of my grandfather.'

I hadn't been expecting this. I was surprised, my heart started to speed up, my hands began to sweat. Oh no, tears were coming, with everyone's gaze on me. No, I wanted to keep my composure, I needed to, I was a doctor for God's sake.

I reacted to the boy's speech with emotion but kept my composure. I was feeling gratitude and respect for him, his future and his family. I know I should have said something, but I just could not. I should have replied,

'Thank you. I am grateful for your grandfather' recovery, but also for his family's support throughout. What saved him were the correct actions of each expert at the right time, along with the family's constant support.'

Dear Melo, medicine has been successful. We all did our job! Attention, availability, collaborative work within the realm of abilities and expertise were the winning mix.

Following the speech, thankfully, the laughter, joy, singing and drinking came back with a vengeance. The celebration for the newlyweds carried on for another day, another night and another day. The religious event was pronounced at the Cathedral of our Lady of the Assumption. There were many occasions to be emotional, joyful and happy. Colourful clothes were to be worn, Celtic beauty was shown, along with youth, intergenerational connections and commitments, flirting, love and joy. A lot was said. Laughter and joy animated everyone. Music and songs were heard. A drone equipped with a camera flew above us to record this moment in the life of this twenty-first century Celtic family of heroes for eternity.

I thought of grandchildren from everywhere in the world. I was content to have been part of this one's life. I know, he will undertake many journeys and experiences, and furthermore, he will always remember that one day his beloved grandfather was saved by the doctor.

And Kevin, the man with Celtic genes, will sing again and again, for a long time."

Silence settled at The Mirage. It was 11.45!

Melo said, "Thank you doctor. Another good story. I shall do the write-up in a few days. By the way, Elpis, would you like to see what I have done so far?"

The doctor replied, "When it is all finished, but do not worry, this writing is first for you."

"Thank you, Doctor. Understood."

Cliff's lookalike walked down the olive tree alley. When Melo saw him, she packed eagerly. She was on time. Melo and her mother met as agreed. They both had a traditional pub lunch on the terrace bordered by a low brick wall. Melo chose a dry-aged sirloin of Owton's beef, and her mother had a crackling roast loin of South Coast pork. Mother and daughter shared a magnificent apple and blackberry crumble with vanilla ice cream to finish off with a peppermint tea. At 3 pm, they made their way to Heathrow airport. Her father was full of joy seeing his family again. They had a lot to tell. At home, he gave his daughter a Nikko metronome and a Zen meditative bell which reminded Melo of her favourite scene from Rick's documentary called *Baraka*. A Zen Buddhist monk was filmed making his way across a town square, clearing his space with the sound of the bell, one small step at a time, each movement, no matter how small, carefully planned and executed with deliberate slowness. Which each step, he was fully in the moment and in the world. Passers-by were walking with respect and *omoiyari*.

Her mother got a jade green and blue Komon kimono and an invitation to go to the Tokyo Olympic Games next summer. Both women were thrilled, everyone was happy and fully conscious of being blessed with life.

*Into whatever houses I enter, I will go into them
for the benefit of the sick*

HIPPOCRATES

Saturday Eight

Autumn was coming. The night before the ninth Saturday, and for the second time, Melo fell asleep in front of her laptop. The girl woke up with yesterday's music in her mind and ears, both eardrums buzzing. She stayed in bed, half-asleep. Brian, the drummer, had driven Melo back home. As usual, the young man had kept silent nearly all the way back home, Amenra, his preferred band of the moment, playing in the background.

Melo liked the song *I saw distance in your eyes*. She talked with enthusiasm and many words to Brian about the video of the song. She felt she could share with him her artistic impressions. Melo felt good in Brian's presence, she could talk to him about her feelings and impressions. From the start, there had been something untold between the two. After rehearsals, Brian and Melo often ended up together, away from the others and comfortably sharing the silence. Neither Brian nor Melo had ever tried cocaine or even alcohol and always retired a couple of metres from the joyful others to be with their respective smartphones, laughing slightly when the others did, just to be part of it all.

Melo admired Brian's drumming skills and, on some occasions, felt they were both playing in harmony. She liked looking at a video with him on his Samsung phone and simply enjoyed listening to his stories about his dog. Brian was a dog lover, just like Booth Cliff in *Once upon a time in Hollywood*. Melo thought he may be autistic too, but maybe not. It did not matter really. Autism was no more a big deal in her life. She felt close to Brian, that was her reality. This feeling seemed to be a bit like with Mia. However ….

At the sound of the alarm, Melo woke up with the memory of last night. Brian had been driving the white Ford Transit Welfare, eyes fixed on the road ahead. She remembered talking about Amenra's music and one fleeting moment of wanting to kiss him. The want was for an instant, ephemeral but strong until it evaporated as fast as it had come.

She remembered. At her home's gate, Melo had got out of the car, bundled up in her blue faux fur trim hood, and looking just like her Baby Yoda sticker, faced the car and waved goodbye. She did not remember going to bed though.

Melo reached for her iPhone. 5.40 am, time to wake up, no time for daydreaming. She got ready and left home at 6.13 am. Her parents were away for the weekend. She opened the door and walked with resolution across the front garden. The Japanese maple tree's leaves were turning to flame. Autumn was coming, and Melo liked it. On the street, she walked down Richmond Avenue towards the underground station. 6.15 am, the road was nearly silent. One could hear the gathering swallows twitter in the sky. A rainbow of fall leaves was appearing in front of Melo's eyes with yellow, brown and magenta leaves blowing joyously about.

Melo was delighted and fully awake despite yesterday's music session, the buzz in her ears and the consequent physical and mental exhaustion.

She arrived at the station. Oyster card out of the pocket a few seconds before arrival at the underground gates, a touch of the contactless card to the yellow reader, gate open.

In the tube, Melo opened *Asclepius: The God of Medicine*, but then closed it as she remembered. She reached her backpack to take another book: *The Soviet Space Dogs* by Olesya Turkina she bought last week at Daunt Books, not far from Harley Street. Sitting comfortably in the nearly empty carriage, Melo admired the many illustrations. She stopped on one page with a photo of a female physician holding a breathing apparatus over the nose of a dog. In her mind was Brian and his habit of scrolling through his dog photos. Then, still staring at the breathing apparatus in the book, the memory of Kevin saved by Dr. Elpis came back to her. She tried to imagine the man who survived with a coil in his brain, under the skull, just as the train stopped at Oxford Circus Station.

6.40 am, walking up the escalator, looking at more illustrations. Overground, a few people around. Melo sensed the *omoiyari* feeling, along with a mixture of joy, contentment and peace. Melo felt close enough to other people to feel joy and respect for others but far enough away to feel free, secure and independent. *Omoiyari* in all its glory.

Walking along Liberty, then Little Marlborough Street, she passed two homeless men still sleeping and dreaming. No coin to give, she felt sorry to miss an opportunity to help. She kept walking, her cheeks now red, ashamed of herself. The magic feeling of before had gone. She entered The Mirage, hunched over, her face hidden behind her golden bouncing curls.

Mia, behind the bar, did not think anything of it and kept swiping her Tinder matches, distributing likes. Love was in the air. At the sight of Melo, she just raised her small, perky nose, and with her intense blue-eyed gaze, looked at the girl and said,

"Hi, I'll bring your matcha tea. By the way, you didn't come last week, you should have told me. The doctor didn't tell me either, only my boss."

"Sorry, Mia, I missed you. I'm here today though."

"And your bike?"

"Not today."

Mia went off and sent her friend a disappointed emoji.

Dr. Elpis was sitting at the back of The Mirage in front of her cappuccino.

Melo pulled the Moleskine notebook and the box from her bag, her face still hidden behind her long hair. She knew that the doctor wouldn't take any notice of her bad mood and would leave her alone with her state of mind which was already changing anyway. Eventually, she said,

"Good morning, Dr. Elpis, how are you going to approach today's subject?"

"I have been hesitating for several weeks, until I thought of one other medical emergency. It happened outside my office, in the underground.

A man had a seizure while travelling.

Immediately, two doctors rushed to help. I was one of them but, following this incident, I carried on with my journey to work, saw patients in Harley Street, then ran back home to face another unpredictable encounter.

Let me tell you.

First, I will share with you one thought I have had for several years. I have been wondering, with my twentieth century rational mind, if Hippocrates would care for a patient ill in the street or not. In the 5th century before Christ, there was no hospital. People were treated in their home or in the temples. My question has been: Did Hippocrates ignore sufferers he was not called to help by a third party in the first place? Were homeless people being cared for? Was anyone falling ill in the street cared for just there, on the street? Or were people kind enough to bring any sick person into a home, to look after him or her and then call the doctor?

To address these questions, I shall refer to ancient texts and make some degree of assumption.

According to Homer, Odysseus wore torn and ragged garments to fool his enemies as a trick to be allowed into his own home by his rivals, who had taken over the place in his long absence. Odysseus was invited to stay in one corner of the dining room, while his enemies were feasting and laughing about him, the newcomer and homeless they erroneously thought him to be. Odysseus, disguised as a tramp, was given food and was involved in discussions and jokes with the people around him. He was cared for.

According to historians, Homer's story depicted the traditional way of dealing with the homeless in the antique Greece. Xenia, the concept of hospitality, applied to beggars too! And the god Zeus Xenios was there to bother! The community was caring in its own way for the homeless but what about the doctors?

We do not know.

What we do know was that Hippocrates cared for people when he was called for in people's homes or temples and did not intervene on his own accord.

Our twenty-first century London is not comparable! Zeus Xenios is no more, there is no ritual to welcome a beggar into a home, solitude has spread with half of London's citizens living alone, and doctors seldom venture out to visit patients in their homes. Doctors act in clinics, hospitals or outside.

The patient is treated on the spot when needed, or in hospitals where clinical evidence, efficiency and rationalisation have all blurred the moral fundamentals of medical care.

Everything today is about 'Right here. Right now.'

In that context, medical emergencies are positively dealt with, all over London and beyond. Defibrillators are everywhere. Patients can be saved from cardiac arrest but also major injuries with ruptured kidneys, brain haemorrhages, broken limbs, attempted suicide, asthma attacks, or even strokes, etc.

And as we humans of the twenty-first century all know, medical emergencies happen across all walks of life and at any moment.

So, let me tell you about the man who suffered an epileptic fit in the London Underground and how I, along with another doctor, did not think twice about running to attend to the sick.

It was in 2006, the year the whale I called Mocha Dick died in the Thames. A few months following the sad event, I was travelling by tube from my home in Pimlico, where I lived before Fitzrovia.

I was in the underground, just three stations away on the Victoria Line. Pimlico, Green Park and Oxford Circus, a six-minute ride. It was 7.45 am. I was sitting in a four-seater area in a carriage, translating some French poetry and lyrics by Michel Houellebecq.

Two seats away, a man became agitated. Passengers around him moved away as one.

Prints of lyrics and poems still in hand, I instantly understood. The man was convulsing. He was having an epileptic fit. His body was agitated with widespread, violent, involuntary contractions. Limbs stiffened and jerked. However, he was unconscious. He had a generalised tonic-clonic seizure or a convulsion, just like Kevin had in my office.

Convulsion is the result of an abnormal unregulated electrical discharge, likened by scientists to a brainstorm, that occurs within the brain and which transiently interrupts normal brain function. As a result, the electrical brainstorm causes altered awareness along with convulsion.

In 2006, I, along with my colleagues and scientists, did not have a clue on how a seizure happened out of the blue, without a brain's physical insult such as a brain haemorrhage or tumour.

However, despite not knowing the *primum movens* of epilepsy, doctors developed efficient treatments in the sixties which are still in use today. These treatments work for most patients but only if taken regularly and at the correct dosage, two fundamentals difficult to achieve today as the result of miscommunication between doctors and patients.

Sadly, in 2006 and even now, miscommunication was due to a lack of care, social issues and solitude. Many epileptics are undertreated, and more seizures are happening with more sudden deaths from epilepsy than ever before in the United Kingdom.

But, let's get back to the convulsing man on the Victoria Line.

The train arrived in Green Park where someone pulled the alarm.

I rushed to help and shouted, 'I'm a doctor.'

At the same time, a young man did exactly the same, and we shouted in concert, 'I'm a doctor.' He reached the convulsing man first, just two seconds before me. The patient was not responding. He was unconscious, eyes and body agitated by a succession of fits. No one was near him; people had already vacated the surrounding area. The attending doctor started the processes which save lives and prevent injuries.

The convulsing patient was turned over by the doctor into the recovery position. Next, he tilted the head to open the airways and prevent suffocation. Breathing and circulation were both checked according to medical precepts. From my colleague's attitude, I understood he did not want me to interfere. He actually did not need any help, was obviously eager to do this, eager to be the hero and the doctor who saved the man in the underground.

I assessed the situation quickly, was further reassured that the paramedics were coming and that yes, there was no need for two doctors to be around. So I carried on my journey to Harley Street, quickly putting out of my mind what had happened and just focussing on the day ahead in my practice.

I arrived at the office at 8.45 am, a few things to sort out before my consultation. I saw one couple that day who always remind me of the famous Terentius Neo fresco from Pompeii. The same connivance between the two, the obvious gender and social equality, even some physical resemblance.

So I saw this couple and said, like always,

'Good morning, Mr. and Mrs. White. What can I do for you today?'

'Dr. Elpis, my nights are so disturbed that we now sleep in different rooms. After fifty years sharing the same bed, it's difficult, you know. Sometimes, I just sit in his room to hear his breathing. The sound of it calms me down and helps me get back to sleep, but on a chair and not by the side of my husband. Doctor, can you help me to get back to a normal night's sleep? Can you help me to get back to sleep by his side?'

While his wife was speaking and complaining, Mr. White remained quiet, his hands resting on the golden fox head moulded as the top of his walking stick, his eyes half-closed. I could see his gentle, wise smile on his face.

I could not come up with a cure for her disturbed sleep though, but in some way I felt reassured that these two people had a powerful emotional link which was only getting stronger with the years passing by. They were caring for each other.

Following this consultation, I carried on working.

And the day developed.

5 pm, time to go back home. I changed into running clothes, put on my Asics shoes and pulled on my Sweaty Betty hat. Twelve more weeks until the London marathon.

In my running gear, I left Harley Street, a small Deuter Speed city backpack fixed around my torso, the Sony sport earphones in my ears, their black wire under the vest running from my ears to the green iPod on the waistband of my trousers. Here I was, out the door of 2000 Harley Street, a quick right turn to Devonshire Street, crossing Marylebone Village and, in a few minutes, I was in Manchester Street.

Fat Boy Slim and its big beat genre music in my ears.

The winter was not far, days were getting shorter and shorter. It was already dark! I was aware of my pineal gland, deep in the brain. It started to produce melatonin, the hormone which mediates dark signals and provides night information to the brain and body. Fifteen minutes later, the endorphins, the human brain's naturally occurring opiates, kicked in, adding their positive effect to the melatonin rush. I felt elated.

Crepuscular darkness was settling, and my brain was aware of the phenomenon despite the artificial light, thanks to the melatonin, and of course my eyes. Every part of my body and brain were functioning in resonance with the ecosystem.

Entering Hyde Park, I made a last-minute decision and altered my routine to run that evening alongside the Serpentine Road rather than through the park. The area appeared too sparsely lit by the artificial light. Running along the Serpentine Road should be safer in this settling darkness.

But to my surprise, at that very moment, a fox. The wild London animal emerged out of a bush and ran towards me. The gaze of the wild animal and mine met. It turned its head towards me, fixed my gaze without flinching, while pursuing its path towards the next bush. I gazed in return and followed my own path. I felt its eyes both vulnerable and revealing; the fox could have seen the same. In that fleeting moment, in that very fraction of a second, I was sharing my wilderness with the London fox. A cerebral interaction between two mammals, with mirrored neurones firing in both brains at the same moment. I felt the connection with the wild animal, equal to equal for one instant.

At the end of the day, the fox was a Londoner just like me. I was running free and safe in Hyde Park, just as this fox was. And that was right in many ways.

I must admit though that I felt euphoric, happy to connect with the animal and its world, a world which was also mine.

I ran with the heartening feeling of contentment and elation, probably supported by the release of dopamine adding its effects to both endorphins and melatonin. One could say I felt the earth happy under my feet and the crystalline air delighted to caress my face. I was feeling the moment with both brain and body, through the limbic and pre-frontal areas of my brain. At that very moment neither the past nor the future mattered. Everything was right here, right now. Life in all of its beautiful simplicity, right here, right now.

I looked at the artificial lights east of the Serpentine. They were exquisitely familiar, Fat Boy Slim's music in my ears.

Just pure emotional rewilding in the middle of twenty-first century London. It was wonderful.

Once home, time for a quick shower before heading to the kitchen. Not enough. My mind wandered. I thought of the young doctor attending to the epileptic patient that morning in the underground. He was probably talking about his exploit to his young wife by now, as he should.

'Today, I saved a man in the underground'. I felt in a way glad he made it before me. I have treated so many patients with seizures in the past, I knew too well how simple it was. It was time for me to leave the youngest to apply their skills and shine.

The doctor carried on speaking.

Then, I sat down and let it go.

In the space of few minutes, Hippocrates and I were talking in the cosy sitting room.

I read Houellebecq's poetry aloud, Hippocrates plays music with his kithara. The whole atmosphere was calming and allowed the emotions and the intellects to collide in peace. Hippocrates said,

'Tell me, Elpis, my sister in the profession. You have explained to me, and I understand that skills and technology are both available to help someone convulsing, but also make the heart beat again, the lung breathe, the kidney filter.

I also understand electricity as a basic part of nature. I comprehend it is a set of physical phenomena associated with the presence and motion of matter that has a property of electric charge.

But does the electricity spread from the brain to the muscles, and if so, how? Tell me how a seizure and convulsion happen.'

I curl up on the sofa, soothed by the music and the tones of my forefather's voice expressing kind and pragmatic words.

'Dear master, scientists and doctors still have not fully explained the propagation of the electricity in epilepsy. We actually still do not understand the exact occurrence or even phenomenon behind it.'

Hippocrates strummed the strings of the kithara with his slender fingers. I said,

'The idea that the mind is a computational system, the computational theory of the mind has simply failed to relate the physiological aspects of the brain's activity to the epilepsy phenomenon. We are still not able to explain why and how a seizure starts and how it spreads. The computational theory has also failed to fully relate the secretion of hormones and the feelings to the brain's functioning to the electrical occurrence. The brain functions are non-linear. More scientists are working away from the computing theory. Our brain cannot be compared to a computer because of its chaotic. These scientists are now using complex mathematical tools to apprehend the non-linear, often chaotic brain and body functions, and may soon gain more understanding of epilepsy and other neurological conditions.'

Music is played and listened to, my body relaxes, and a feeling of contentment prevails, in spite of the complex questioning. And I thought, the mathematicians may one day explain epilepsy fully.

Even though humanity will still need the help and the experience of the clinicians, the ones who directly observe, care for the patient and act right here, right now."

Silence settled in The Mirage. After a few minutes, Melo said,

"Thank you so much for today's stories. Doctor, are you still running?"

"Not anymore. I lost the will, really. I have to admit though that each time I see a good runner, I get an intense nostalgic feeling and just feel the urge to run with him or her."

"I understand. I feel the same at the sight of a cyclist, I just feel the urge to follow and cycle with a good cyclist."

"You see Melo, this is empathy. You have it! Your brain secretes oxytocin when it is required!"

The blogger did not reply but let a big smile invade her beautiful face.

Then, Elpis reached for her bag to take out a piece of paper. This is for you, a copy of the translation of Michel Houellebecq's poem *Isolement*."

"I have to go, Dr. Elpis. I have to be with Brian in just one hour for a studio session in Clerkenwell."

"Who is Brian?"

"The band's drummer. We will play our first gig next Saturday, so much to do, you know. See you next week."

Melo packed her Moleskine notebook and the box with the three pens in it with care. She left the doctor with an "*Au revoir*," and walked down the corridor.

Mia left what she was doing and came to Melo. "Let's go to the Crocobar. Tuesday night?"

Melo froze and took a few seconds to reply, "Yes, why not, 6 pm?"

"Sounds good. I will wait for you near the Rags and Bones."

"Sure, see you then."

"Goodbye, see you then."

Melo left in a hurry. Sitting in the underground, as she took her book out of her backpack, she noticed Elpis' sheet of paper. She read:

ISOLEMENT Isolation, Houellebecq, translated by me, 2018

Where am I?
Who are you?
What am I doing here?
Take me with you anywhere
Anywhere but not here
Help me to forget
All I have been
Can you create my past?
Can you give meaning to the night
Can you create the sun?
And the appeased Dawn
No, I am not sleepy
I will kiss you
Are you my friend?
Do answer me, answer me
What am I?
There is fire everywhere
I do not hear any noise
I am maybe crazy
I need to lie down
And sleep a little bit
I may try
To clean my eyes
Tell me who I am
And look at my eyes
Are you my friend?
Will you make me happy?
The night is not finished
And the night is in fire
Where is heaven?
Where the gods have gone?

PROLOGUE

Parenthese

Melo and Mia meeting in Soho

Tuesday night in Soho. 5.55 pm. Mia was standing by the window of Rags and Bones, swiping through Tinder and Facebook.

Melo recognised Mia from afar, smiled and walked decisively towards her friend, back straight, shoulders back, curls bouncing like a veil in front of her green eyes.

6 pm. "Hi Melo, let's go, the Crocobar is just around the corner in Manette street."

The two girls walked side by side till they reached their destination. On arrival, Mia opened the black painted door fully covered with punk stickers. Considerately, she let Melo go in first. The bar was just to the left of the entrance. Two waitresses, a gothic girl and a rock guy, were talking to two boldly pierced old punks.

Mia gazed at Melo, who seemed to be daydreaming behind her curls. "What do you want to drink? I don't think they've got matcha tea here you know."

Melo did not reply.

Mia then addressed the gothic girl; "One Peroni and one Coke please." She paid with a touch of her Samsung wallet, took the two glasses, and said, "Let's move to the back."

Melo followed her friend, curls bouncing and safely covering her young face.

The backroom was dimly lit; all was dark apart from the white painted skull on the back wall. Mia found a table in the northwest corner. The duo sat down.

Pretty Vacant was playing. *Too much is illusions,* something like that.

Mia took her bottle, gazed at Melo's green eyes and, with a determined and friendly tone, said, "Cheers Melo, welcome to the Crocobar!"

With a gentle head tilt, Melo moved the curls away, took the can of coke with a faint hesitation, smiled like a clown and clanged Mia's bottle, hard, with her own.

"Cheers."

Mia was surprised at the violent impact and was nearly ready to tell Melo off, but she didn't say anything. The two sipped, gazing at each other. Then, Mia took her Galaxy Samsung and started to type frenetically, with her thumb moving and touching rhythmically and at high speed across the screen.

Melo took her iPhone from her backpack and asked,

"Do you know where the toilets are?"

"Just downstairs."

Melo put the phone back in the bag and stood up with the can of coke in her hand.

"Leave your drink here, I'll keep it safe, don't worry."

"Ok."

Melo went down the very old and tiny wooden stairs. The toilets were opposite. They were small, no room to leave a bag or a can really.

However, she managed, and went back upstairs.

"I never saw such a tiny bathroom."

"You should never bring your drink into a bar or restaurant's bathroom. And never leave your drink unattended. Someone could put a tablet in it, you know. It's called a spike and will make you weird and unwell. Don't ever get spiked, Ok?"

Four post-punk girls came in. They were all giggling but one. At first sight, Mia didn't like her. The girl was gazing persistently at Melo, obviously interested. But moreover, she seemed to be a bully and was obviously looking for someone to hurt. Melo was looking at the screen of her iPhone and listening to Machine Death's bass playing from the jukebox.

Mia said, "Do you smoke?"

"No."

"Never mind, let's get out of here."

Mia stood up and left. Melo followed quietly.

Outside of the Crocobar, Mia leaned on the wall, took out her Blue American Spirit organic tobacco. Melo stood by her side, backpack well-positioned, eyes fixed on the iPhone.

Mia skilfully rolled a cigarette, lit it, and said, "Let's go to Soho Park. I don't like this place."

Melo carefully put the phone in her coat's side pocket and followed her friend without a word. She'd been interested in the music at the Crocobar, but now she was feeling uneasy.

On the way, Mia stopped at a corner shop, asked for four cans of beer and two Mars bars.

The duo walked the Soho Street maze, going on and off the pavements, weaving around the crowds of joyful drinking people of all kinds. Everybody was out to have fun. At the park, Mia chose a well-lit spot not far from the Twentieth Century Fox building. She then diligently put two plastic bags down on the grass and said,

"Let's sit down here."

Mia sat in a lotus position, and Melo on her tailbone, hugging her folded legs, the backpack still on.

Mia said, "Cool, we can relax now. Cheer up." She took two cans of beers, opened one and gave it to Melo. She then took another can and added, "Cheers."

And again, Melo banged her friend's drink too hard and with a big smile, as if it was forced, though it was not. Melo was happy.

Mia said, "You know these punk girls were there for a fight. Did you see how the one with pink hair was looking at you?"

"Which girls?"

"In the Crocobar, just near us. You didn't see them? You are a daydreamer, you really are." She then took a sip of beer, and added, "So, Melo, do you like boys or girls?"

"Yes, I do."

"I mean, do you have a boyfriend or a girlfriend?"

"Oh, I don't, I don't know."

"What do you mean, you don't know?

"I've never kissed anyone. I do not feel like it really."

Mia looked at Melo, asking herself if the girl was dumb, a dumb nerd, or just a rich immature kid with no common sense.

"You've never been kissed?"

"What did you say?"

"Kiss someone?"

"No, never."

"Do you miss it?"

"Not really. You know I'm autistic, maybe that's why."

"I have a neighbour back home who is autistic, he is so weird, you know? Much more than you are. Melo, I have read somewhere that some people do not need sex. They are called asexual. You may be one of them."

"I feel close to you, Mia, and I trust you. Maybe you can guide me."

"Melo, I only like boys. What about your friends, have you ever experienced ... flirting?"

"I do not have friends apart from you."

Mia was taken aback. Why was she always talking about autism?

"I heard you play music with a band."

"Yes."

"So you have friends."

"Yes, Jaz is cool, he is the leader and singer. Zoltan is nice too. And Brian, the drummer, is a South Londoner like me. He lives in Putney and always drives me back home in the band's Ford Transit Welfare."

"Did you ever hang out with one of them?"

"What do you mean?"

"Don't worry. So much to learn. Melo, I can help you create a Tinder profile. Let's take some photos."

"Thanks for the idea, but I don't like photos. And I want to remain anonymous on the internet. That is my number one rule in life. I don't have any accounts or subscriptions, apart from my blog."

"I understand. That's alright, I guess. Let me show you my matches, you may find one of them attractive."

Mia opened Tinder and swiped through her sixty-six matches. Melo just saw one human being after another, with nothing to catch her interest, until the twelfth profile.

"I like his name. Keanu. It's cool." Mia kept swiping, then Melo said, "I have written a poem for you, Mia, can I read it?"

"Yes, please."

Mia miia, My Mia

Sitting outside The Mirage

Mia miia, My Mia,

One blue denim leg across the other

Mia miia, My Mia

A blue camel between two snow white fingers

Mia miia, My mia,

The other thumb touching the screen

Blue eyes seeping through

Her very own world

Mia, miia, My Mia,

Tick tick, ticking the likes

Pretty perky nose reddish by the candy snow

Mia, miia, My Mia

Dressed in her virtual bubble

A plane tracing the purple sky

Above My Mia, Mia my Miia

"Oh that is cool."

The girls giggled.

"That is really cool. I like it. However, I don't smoke blue camels, and don't do drugs either. And … and my name is not Mia. You and the doctor have called me Mia from the beginning, but it's not my name."

"Yes, you told me that before. Remind me, what's your real name?"

"Catalina Maria Dona Porcel. My father chose that name. It was because of his admiration of Goya, the painter. My name is derived from his famous painting Dona Isabel De Porcel. When my father left Ethiopia, his country, in 1991, he tried to carry on painting and got an interest in Goya and his way of depicting human cruelty."

Melo wondered, "Who first called you Mia?"

"I don't know, I cannot remember. The point is, Mia is not my name."

To which Melo replied, "I'm not called Melo either!"

Silence settled between the two. Mia reached for the blue American tobacco, the Rizla paper and the extra slim filters, then said,

"If we are going to be friends, we should know each other's real names, shouldn't we?"

Melo gazed intensely at Mia and replied.

"I agree. Let's keep them secret though."

Mia rolled a cigarette with skill and care, raised her head, and gazed at her friend.

"My name is F(-)"

"Nice to know you F(-), Melo, I want to be your friend forever."

Mia laid down the cigarette to embrace her new friend. Melo, still tightly holding her thighs, gently rocked towards Mia and the two relaxed, holding each other's bodies tight, Melo's head on her one and only new friend's shoulder.

Mia murmured Billy's *Bad Guy* song. "Too doot, too doot. I'm the ..."

Melo listened to Mia, feeling the comfort of her presence and the warmth of another human body.

The night settled in Soho Square. Mysterious encounters happened in the unknown and around the two.

Yet, it seemed to Melo that only both of them were in the square.

Mia showed Melo photos of her paintings on her Samsung phone. Mia loved watercolour painting, that was her passion. Melo nodded, drank more and made funny smirks and grimaces. Melo told Mia loudly about being an anthropologist and could not stop laughing when Mia tried to repeat the word. Mia kept looking at her paintings and told her that she wanted to find the perfect red colour on snow for one of her painting projects with an injured eagle in the mountain. Melo giggled and giggled.

The girls drank more, Melo for the first time ever. Both giggled and giggled. Melo talked louder, enjoying the night to her core.

She took her phone and chose *You'll be a woman soon* from her Spotify list. Both girls listened to Marco's sensual and sweet melody three times. Mia had her hand resting on her friend's shoulder, her side and breast ever so close to Melo's back. The two young women felt comfortable and happy to be together, sang with Marco, giggled and giggled.

It was as if they grew closer, became almost sisterly, as they listened to the melody. With no further talk, Melo then selected on Youtube The showdown of the House of Blue Leaves, and then without intermission, her preferred scene, the fight between the Bride and O-Ren-Ishii. Melo and Mia both knew the film well and seemed to agree about and enjoy the same bits.

Mia kept murmuring, "Yes, cool, whoo, that is nuts, wicked," and so on and so forth. Melo nodded first when she saw the whirling axe and when Uma ran up the banister like a funambulist after having fought so well and dismembered so many with her sword. What a performance! The duo admired the end of the fight scene with reverence, where the courage and fighting skills of the two women were equally valued by Tarantino. Melo and Mia knew well that The Bride and O-ren-Ishii both deserved revenge, but only one could win. That was real life. One had to die, but with dignity. A moment of sadness was shared at the sight of the awful O-Ren-Ishii's death, even though it was not the first time they'd seen her half-beheading in the exquisite snowy Japanese garden.

Melo felt mellow and enjoyed the physical closeness of Mia. She felt she liked her. Was that real friendship?

An UberX car booked by Mia arrived with a drop-off estimate in Richmond of £23.33. Once Melo was securely in the car, Mia waved goodbye and went on all alone, walking tall to her destiny.

Melo fell asleep in the car with the lyrics of the flower of carnage in her head …

I will abstain from every voluntary act of mischief and corruption; and, further from the seduction of females or males, of freemen and slaves

HIPPOCRATES

Saturday Nine

Melo woke up late on Saturday the 13th of October. The band had played a gig, the first for many months. The crowd was just great, the mosh pit cathartic, and the music sounded good to Melo. Everyone followed the bass. Melo was exhausted though. Following the show, she found it hard to have to pack and keep a smile for everyone after such intense music.

The girl had realised yesterday how physically demanding metal music was and concluded that she would never play professionally. The whole experience was strenuous, she felt. However, the music was intense, and Brian was great. She remembered catching a glance of him through her curls while playing. His silver chain was glittering, and the wolf tattooed on his right shoulder looked animated, expressing its wildness so intensely that Melo had to gaze at it while playing. She remembered. At the end of the gig, Brian stood and unfolded his body away from the double bass drums and cymbals. Melo felt at that precise moment the urge to hold him tight in a big hug, rest her head on his chest, mixing both of their sweat and their body heat. But it did not happen, it was just a feeling of a fleeting moment. The band packed in silence, while the crowd around was noisy and happy. They drove back home in the Ford Transit Welfare filled with the material and instruments. Brian broke the silence and said,

"Have you ever been up Primrose Hill?"

"No, never."

"Melo, let's go there next week, it's just a few minutes away from here."

"Ok."

Brian stopped the van at the traffic light, turned and gazed at Melo with a big smile. Orange light, the drummer's foot pressed on the clutch, the palm of his hand gently pushing against the gear stick spring. Brian faced the road in front, the big smile still on his face, Amenra, his preferred band of the moment, playing in the background, French words, *dans mon coeur j'emporterai… je te cherche … désespérence….*

When they arrived at Melo's home, she got out of the car, bundled up in her blue faux fur trim hood, and, just like her Baby Yoda sticker, gazed at Brian and waved goodbye. She did not remember going to bed though, she'd simply reached the dreaming world as soon as she hit the pillow.

The next day, Melo grasped her iPhone. No time to waste. She could not be late.

In one movement, she was up. Melo took the phone and plugged it into its charger.

Now brushing her teeth, then, instinctively, she gently brought her free hand to her stomach, covered the belly button with the tip of her thumb, spread the hand kindly over her body, her middle finger fiddling with the soft hair down there. The young woman felt the natural heat of her body and imagined she was holding her Baby Yoda lookalike womb. It was a good feeling.

She put on her jeans and top. A quick look at the weather app. Today, rain, most of the day. Okay. Let's get ready. She grabbed her laptop and put it in the backpack, already filled with books and her precious pen box. Melo went downstairs.

"Darling Melo, have a cup of tea, I've just made one for you."

"No, Mother, I'm already late."

"Don't forget your umbrella, it's raining."

"Ok, see you later. I should be back before midday I think, I need some rest."

"Grandma will be here."

"Oh great, see you later."

Melo loved her grandmother; the old woman was so special to her. Her French accent had always been so special to Melo.

Outside, the rain was pouring down. The weeping Japanese maple tree was standing, its palm-like leaves fighting against the repetitive attacks of the rain, drop after drop. Melo walked with care under the black umbrella. With a graceful movement, she kicked a plastic bag in the middle of the pavement, thinking of the one responsible for her grandmother's hip fracture last year. Since that incident, the old woman had not been the same, just repeating the same questions on and on, and using more French words than ever before.

At the station, Oyster card out of the pocket a few seconds before arrival at the underground gates, a touch of the contactless card to the yellow reader, gate open.

The train journey was quick today, as Melo slept at some point on the way.

Going up Oxford Circus station's escalator, Melo took out her umbrella. When she came out of the tube station, the rain was still pouring down. Melo's eardrums were buzzing with last night's music. She opened her umbrella, looked at the circus, waiting for the positive sign on the traffic light. The green man light came. In one movement, she ran the diagonal path of the hybrid Shibuya-Oxford Circus crossing, thinking of The Bride gliding up the staircase with her sword dripping blood. Brian's naked, wet chest from yesterday came to her mind too.

She kept running. Melo found something special, something elating about running in the rain holding an umbrella overhead. She loved it. Nothing was awkward. She was not too tall actually. Melo was feeling good in and out of her body. She was a happy young woman in the midst of rainy London.

Seven minutes later, there she was at The Mirage, her cheeks and the tip of her nose bright red, the bottom of her mac and her trainers all wet.

"Good morning, Melo. Let me take your umbrella and coat. Elpis is waiting for you."

"Thank you, Mia, you are so good to me."

Mia winked at her and replied, "No prob, you are my favourite customer, you know. A wicked one though."

Melo kissed her friend's cheek and walked down the dimly lit passage.

"Hi Melo, good morning. What ghastly weather, is it not?"

"Not too bad. I like the rain, you know? I feel tired though, we played our first gig yesterday. It was good. But I am just exhausted, and my ears are still buzzing."

Melo sat down as she realised how cool Dr. Elpis was today. Bright red nails, just like her mother's with her 'scandalous' polish, a black hoody, black, shiny skinny-legged jeans and red Doc Martins. All her rings on.

Even with this post-punk allure, uneasiness did not exist around the doctor. Melo had never experienced awkwardness in the presence of Dr. Elpis. It was like the doctor's very existence was soothing. The *omoiyari* feeling was always present around her, compassion too. For Melo, it was like she was free to be, to suffer or not in the presence of the doctor. Melo realised that reality today, probably because of her mindfulness following the crazy run in the rain.

Elpis began, "Melo, have you got a boyfriend?"

That was not expected. Melo was taken aback; she felt almost choked, as if stupefied. She just managed to reply, without thinking straight,

"No, I'm a nerd. I am an autistic nerd, an Asper if you like, and I like to be that way."

Melo felt herself blushing. In a faint head movement, she hid behind her curls and tried to fold her long legs out of the way, feeling uncomfortable in her own body now, not knowing how to position all of it. Behind her curls, she added, "I am autistic, you know."

"Melo, you said that before, but for me, you are a young human being with your own uniqueness, someone who knows how to listen and to write. You are a woman and a friend too."

Elpis knew that Melo was feeling very mild social awkwardness, nothing more. The doctor doubted the diagnosis. Melo was not disabled in any way, on the contrary she was an independent human being who was bettering herself through work and consistency. The

146

doctor also understood that Melo had been fortunate with family support. But in any case, the doubtful diagnosis of autism was one part of the young woman's identity jigsaw. It was precious to her and telling Melo she was not so autistic as she thought would have caused offense. The doctor remained silent, waiting for the discomfort to lessen.

Melo decided to get back some control and said, "What about you, Doctor, are you married?"

"I was once, a long time ago. I love men though! Some are so beautiful, handsome and so special, some are boring, ugly, fat or stupid! However, I love them all. I just love the masculinity, you know. I just could not live without men's company! That would just be hell!

I love humans in general. And this can be complicated for a doctor you know. It can be tricky sometimes. How to deal with unconditional trust along with the nearly constant intimate exposure to another human while working? My profession is in a position of power, you know.

The oath is clear-cut on that subject though. Respect of confidentiality, and also no corruption of any kind. Looking back, I think I have easily worked in accordance with the oath, possibly because I am by nature averse to any use of power for my own self-interest and cannot be corrupted by money. A long time ago though, I must admit that I was once at risk of corruption. Melo, I was about your age, and he was so handsome."

The doctor was intensely aware of Melo's prudishness, and the necessary duty for her to respect it, to be kind to the young adult, her nerdish personality and her conviction of being autistic. She decided, on the spot, to smooth over the atmosphere with a clever diversion.

"Let me tell you a story I have never told before. But let me first talk about mosquitoes in the vicinity of humanity."

Melo opened her Moleskine notebook and wrote at the top of a clear page, 'Mosquitoes in the vicinity of humanity'.

The doctor then said, "I was a young doctor working in Brest, Brittany. I was at the university hospital named La Cavale Blanche, meaning White Escape, on the third floor in the brand-new travel clinic I had helped to set up as part of my studies in Tropical Diseases. The hospital was brand-new too. It had opened just the year before.

On that day, I had to finish the review of the current understanding of dengue fever, a viral infection transmitted to humans by mosquitoes and responsible of yearly epidemics in Asia, Africa and South America.

Like malaria, dengue fever is a human disease carried by mosquito bites. It is responsible for major epidemics and can be fatal for young children, sick people and the elderly.

In the absence of any treatment, teams around the world have been working on the development of a vaccine for many years with little success so far.

I had been asked by the head of the service, Professor Arnaud Cenac to review the current understanding of the disease. In his view, it could soon become a major global issue as the result of global warming and growing cargo traffic. And the future will indeed prove him right!

Today, some twenty years following his prediction, dengue fever is a pandemic affecting more than a hundred countries. About 390 million dengue infections occur every year. Africa, the Americas, the Eastern Mediterranean, Southeast Asia and the Western Pacific regions are currently the most seriously affected. And Europe is now counting a few new cases year by year.

Two mosquitos are responsible for this annual pandemic, *Aedes aegypti* and the Asian tiger mosquito. The female of both live in the vicinity of humans, biting them during the day, drawing, bite by bite, the human blood essential to eggs. Without human blood, *Aedes aegypti* female cannot produce eggs and would simply disappear from Earth.

That is how life is sometimes!

We all depend on each other; the ecosystem is entwined.

Human beings are essential to the *Aedes aegypti* survival. However, the Asian tiger mosquito occasionally bites animals too and in doing

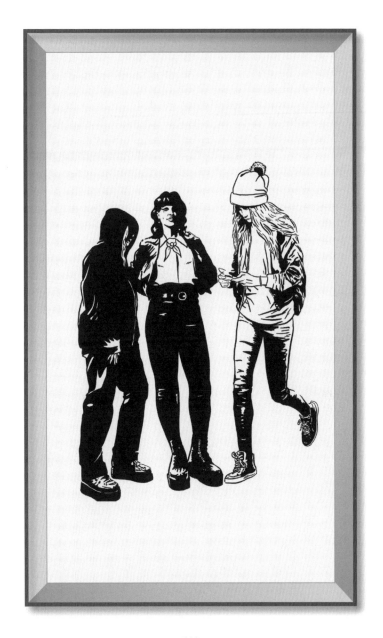

so can transfer disease from animals to humans, like the Zika virus!

The fearless Asian tiger mosquito is an invader too. It originated from Asia but has now invaded the whole world, thanks to cargo traffic. It is listed as one of the one hundred worst invasive alien species with the potential of biting one billion more humans every year by 2050.

The scientists reckon that its world invasion began in the seventeenth century. The mosquito took advantage of worldwide shipping to invade the Americas and other parts of the globe. Climate change and global warming have helped further its settlement all around the world.

As a young doctor, I remember being intrigued by the mosquito's appearance, with its bold, shiny, black scales and distinct silver white scales. The back, called the scutum, is black with the distinguishing white strap down the centre, beginning at the dorsal surface of the head and continuing along the thorax.

The strength and characteristics of its eggs make it a good traveller at sea. The female, well-fed with human blood, lays them on the side of tires. Her eggs then travel all around the world, withstanding desiccation for up to one year! In the eighties, America tried something to stop the invader. The US Authority required all used tires entering the country from known endemic countries to be dry-cleaned and treated with fumigants. However, the invasion was not to be stopped and carried on with the detection of a first specimen in Kent, UK, last year.

Scientists are working on the creation of genetically modified mosquitoes. I am not sure this is a good idea though. The risks attached to genetic manipulation are still unknown. This is another subject of concern I may talk to you about another time.

Let's go back to the year 1996, when Professor Cenac and I became interested in the mosquito and dengue fever.

I was writing, collecting and studying all available data methodically for a few hours before the start of my clinical work.

The first patient entered the room. My mind was still busy with the Asian tiger insect and its danger. I raised my head to be taken aback by the man who just entered the room. My breath was literally taken by the beauty of this man. He was a geologist going to Mali, West Africa, I suddenly remembered from my list. He was dressed casually with jeans and a jumper, nothing special. His hair was long and dark, his wide-set eyes a beautiful hazelnut brown. His demeanour and posture were both attractive too. I was struggling not to be absolutely hypnotised. Following two hours of intellectual work with mosquitoes and dengue fever, I tried and managed, with great difficulty, to concentrate on my doctoring.

At that moment, and in the consulting room of the brand-new hospital, the man needed vaccinations and professional support from a doctor, me. He was going to travel to Mali, where he has been appointed as a geologist for a new mining project. He was going to work in the fields, where all sorts of mosquitoes, parasites and germs were still living in relative peace, away from urbanisation.

However, as soon as the man opened the door of the small hospital room, I froze. I felt buzzing in my ears, my heart beating fast. I was not blushing yet though, but my fingers were already all sweaty. I remember still now, his gentle and kind smile, much like that of the first ever boy I had secretly loved at school. He had an abundance of beautiful dark hair, the colour of a jay's feathers. It was ridiculous and unacceptable for me to feel that way though, I should focus my mind on the work I had to do. So, I got on with work. I asked questions, one after another, about his planned work in Mali, his previous experiences in mining other parts of the world. I had one sole aim: the assessment of his individual infectious risk to establish the best option in terms of vaccinations and malaria prevention.

Thereafter, we discussed dengue fever. The already well-travelled geologist told his concerns about getting it. He'd seen a few colleagues affected by dengue. It was not nice at all and was debilitating for at least two weeks. We then talked about *Aedes aegypti* and its Asian cousin, the tiger mosquito, and their worrying spread worldwide.

'You know, Doctor, I actually fear dengue fever even more than malaria. Will we ever get a vaccine against it?'

'Not yet, I am afraid to say. The dengue virus is very complex, has several variants, and that makes things complicated for the design of a vaccine. However, the drug industry is working at it. So, for now, I will vaccinate you against yellow fever, hepatitis B, hepatitis A, rabies and typhoid.'

In silence, I got ready to proceed with the inoculations.

At my request, the gorgeous man took off his jumper, revealing his beautiful and muscular physique with its perfect, smooth, bare skin, just a few rogue hairs between the stunningly pigmented nipples. Help!

A little voice in my head said, 'A bit of professionalism please, Doctor, do not look that way, please!'

I then tried my best to focus on the various syringes and, one at a time, measured the gauge and delicately pierced the beautiful skin. I gently pushed the shaft of the needle in a smooth movement, then with my right index finger, pushed the syringe's plunger to fully inject the vaccine, all the while talking about dengue fever and the invasion of *Aedes albopictus*, the black and white Asian tiger mosquito. All done!

Things went quickly thereafter. I remember shaking his hand with a feeling of triumph and victory for managing to be a doctor till the end! I also remember his trusting look to me, the professional. I liked it!

Following this hard work to remain professional at all costs, I saw the next patient. She was a lady in her forties, a petite French lady with an elegant, serene, and restrained beauty. She did not speak much but said, rather bluntly,

'I need all the possible vaccines.' The woman told me she was going to travel for a year all around the world. I then asked the purpose of the travel. The lady bluntly replied, 'My family, my husband and my three children died in a road traffic accident six months ago. I have no one left. I have to go away.'

She then froze, looking at me bluntly. She would not show her emotion. I felt it was for her an existential necessity. I understood and shut up. I swallowed my saliva, tried to keep my composure, but then acknowledged the tragedy with probably improper and awkward words and said,

'I am sorry, I understand.' Something like that. Five words, one sentence. Something I often say to invite a kind silence to quiet the emotions and suffering.

Mutely, I wrote something and got prepared.

I vaccinated the woman with all vaccines she may need in her new voyage.

Following this consultation at the brand-new travel clinic, I thought about the diversity of humanity, of its suffering, and the importance of the ecosystem around each human being. I also tried to comprehend the complex interrelationship between all these components.

For several months, I reflected on the necessity for a doctor to always be open-minded, with an available scientific and systematic mind with regard to whatever situation he or she is facing at a particular point of time, to be able to catch Kairos by the hair when needed. And this must happen, even if Eros is at stake. Professionalism and medical ethics are both necessary, even in the fleeting moment. Knowledge is not sufficient. A strong moral attitude is necessary to deal with any of life's possibilities.

Whatever, in connection with my professional practice or not in connection with it, I see or hear in the life of men, which ought not to be spoken of abroad, I will not divulge, as reckoning that all such should be kept secret

HIPPOCRATES

Saturday Ten

Melo and Brian did not go up Primrose Hill in the end. The two completely forgot that Melo would not be playing with the band on that Friday night.

Brian was the first to realise it. He sent Melo a crying skull emoji. To which she replied, 'Sorry, next Friday maybe'. He sent a winking skull, to which she replied with her preferred Baby Yoda sticker.

On that Saturday, Melo woke up at 5.30 am. Her father came upstairs with a cup of tea. He kindly took the laptop off the bed and sat by his daughter's side.

"Time to wake up," he whispered, while caressing Melo's cheek.

She opened her eyes, stretched, and unfolded her body with a big yawn.

In forty-five minutes, she was ready. She grabbed her bike and cycled to Soho.

Mia was outside The Mirage, having a cigarette. Melo turned right, towards the opposite wall. Mia inhaled, savouring the last bit, threw the butt, crushed it with her foot, and walked towards her friend.

"Hi Melo. I managed to read and understand your blog on coworking. Interesting. I enjoyed it. Let me lock up your bike. Looks like there's a scratch just below your name. Next time, I will paint it over if you want."

"Sounds good, Mia." Melo held her friend in a big cuddle before going inside.

"I'll bring your matcha tea."

"Dr. Elpis, good morning. I just came back from four days of coastal walking around Saint Yves. Look, mosquito bites. Do you think the Asian tiger mosquito you talked about last week is responsible for these?"

"I don't think so. That dreaded mosquito has not been reported in the UK this year, I believe. I am sorry for you though, you have got a lot of bites, poor thing."

"I am used to getting them, mosquitoes like me, I guess. Why is that, Doctor?"

"I do not know. Doctors do not understand why some people are more susceptible to mosquito bites than others. We just know that when there are mosquitoes around, some people will be bitten and some not."

"I thought it was something to do with smell."

"That is one theory, but it is just not sufficient, there are other reasons which are still unknown."

"I was with my mother in Saint Yves. She is a walker, you know, she asked me to join her this year. I was reluctant initially. My mother talks all the time, you know. She has never accepted my autism and just does not respect my tendency towards silence. She has a way of always suggesting possible reasons for my differences and this has often annoyed me. It is like she sees my autism as shameful for the family. I have not talked to her about my feelings for years. She thought that was my autism, but it was the way I found to protect myself against her constant questions and assumptions.

This year's walk was good though, and I am glad I went with her. I was more talkative, I guess, and for once, we were connected. I told her about your patient who lost all her family in a single accident. She was shocked by the woman's loss and curious to know what you, the doctor, did. When I told her you just gave all the vaccines you could think of, she did not understand. She told me that you should have checked if she was depressed, proposed some medication or psychotherapy. I did not reply to her, I did not tell about the other bit of the story either. However, I believe that what you did was the right thing.

Doctor, I am thankful to you for revealing a doctor's life to me. I now understand that being simply human is sometimes better medical care than giving tablets or trying to make a diagnosis. I am convinced that the woman of last week's story got some comfort following the meeting with you. You respected her intense pain mixed with a strong volition to go around the world, just go. I am certain you made her stronger with your soft, non-inquisitive care and consideration. I wish all doctors could be like you."

"I guess my profession should always be about trust between two individuals, two autonomous and independent people. The doctor needs to respect the patient's independence and autonomy, even in the adversity. And the patient needs to trust that the doctor will apply his or her skills and knowledge within a defined ethical frame.

Confidentiality, the subject of today's talk, is the major element of that trust relationship. It is a major part of medical ethics. It is important for the patient, but also for the doctor, as he or she needs to be convinced that she has all the information to make a diagnosis.

At the time of the HIV epidemic in Paris and the UK, the notion of confidentiality was tested in a big way. There was a dilemma between containing the epidemic and the social stigma attached to the disease.

Should we signal which patients had HIV in hospital wards? Should we differentiate medical care between HIV patients and others? In France, the medical authorities decided quickly. Things should be kept simple. Any patient was to be treated the same, but doctors and health care associates would have to take precautions to limit the infectious risk for any patient, whatever their condition. The UK went beyond that. It was decided that HIV patients would not be reported by name to the health authorities in respect of their confidentiality and the Hippocratic oath. Patients would be protected from social stigma.

However, and sadly, things have been different for patients with TB, tuberculosis, one other severe infectious disease. The reality even today is that any patient with the condition is reported by name to the health authority. The reporting system helps to contain the infection within the community. However, it adds stigma to the individual affected.

When experts track mosquitos to try to prevent and limit dengue

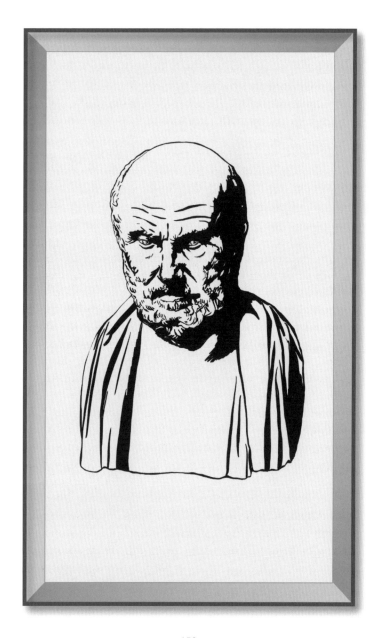

fever outbreaks, doctors and their allies track TB patients and their contacts and meticulously trace close connections one TB patient has had. The knowledge of the whole truth can be vital to contain, prevent, and limit any epidemic. However, social stigma is also at stake and, furthermore, the breach of the oath can then undermine the care of the patient.

Let me tell you.

Tuberculosis was still happening in London at the turn of the twenty-first century. The capital had one of the highest TB rates of any city in Western Europe, you know. Hospital doctors and health carers were working at tracking the disease and treating patients. Public opinion and the media did not care though. I did not care either, until that day.

I was at the Royal Academy of Arts Museum in Burlington House, between the Ritz and Piccadilly Circus. I had been invited for the opening of the exhibition of new landscape works by David Hockney.

At the sight of the oil painting called Woldgate Woods, at its impressive size of 182.9 by 365.8 cm, I was transported, as if by magic, to the Brittany countryside of my childhood and its leafy paths.

While anyone else in the museum could attest that I was in the prestigious London Royal Academy in front of this huge picture, in my mind, I was not. I was somewhere else.

I was back in the Brittany countryside on my very special cherry-red bicycle under the variable leafy green canopies, one or two sun rays darting through on occasion or simply caressing the leaves above me. The tree trunks curtsied one after another at the passage of the mischievous cycling child I used to be. It was pure magic!

This quasi-telepathic transportation into my own past lasted just a few minutes but was physically and emotionally intense, so much so that it felt like an eternity, an eternal spacetime continuum. I was stunned by the joy of being surrounded by such a loving and familiar environment.

Melo, it was more than nostalgia. It was an emotional journey through David Hockney's work of art to my childhood countryside.

The moment was just wholesome and delightful!

I will remember that telepathic transportation at the gallery in front of David Hockney's painting forever and ever. That is for sure!

The next day, I was working when another David called. He wanted to talk about a difficult situation.

He told me, 'Good morning, Doctor, how are you today?'

'I am fine, David, thank you. What can I do for you?'

Still under the spell of Hockney's art, I could have happily spoken about my telepathic transportation experience, but I did not, it was not appropriate. Rather, I reflected. It was unusual for David to ask to talk to me on the phone. I sensed there was something important to be told.

'One of my warehouse agents has been under the weather for several months. He is called Jonathan and has been on and off work with a cough since last September. I just saw him a few minutes ago. Doctor, he is not right, he doesn't look well to me, and his wretched cough will not calm down. This all seems very unusual to me. I am concerned, Doctor. Would you mind seeing him, I do not feel comfortable leaving the poor man working in such a state.'

David kept on talking, saying that Jonathan had gone to A&E and to his GP several times, that he was given various antibiotics and other treatments, the names of which he was unsure of. The man had worked for the company for about two years. He was one of the workers in the large warehouse, where daily goods were received and then sent away. He was a strong and courageous young man, a very good team player too and was appreciated by all. By the tone of voice and the words David chose, I sensed his concerns for his fellow human being. I immediately agreed to see him.

'I understand, I will see Jonathan today at 3 pm. I will help Jonathan and let you know, David.'

3 pm, time to see the first patient of the afternoon. I called the receptionist. 'Can you send the next patient in please.'

Jonathan entered the room. 'Hi, Doc.'

'Good afternoon, please, take a seat. How can I help you today?'

The man was young, muscular and tall, with beautiful short, dark, woolly hair. However, I saw the signs of an underlying disease undermining the luminosity of his youth and strength. The man's skin tone was dull, with sunken eyes, his posture slightly awkward. I could see he was trying to stand politely when he was actually feeling exhausted, his neck muscles stiff, as though getting ready for the next coughing fit. This young man was clearly being eaten away by an underlying disease. I could see it immediately, but I forced myself to be systematic. A doctor should never jump to conclusions but needs to observe, listen, ask the right questions, examine, memorise and think.

He told me, 'I keep coughing, the meds are just not working. I sweat too much, especially at night. I don't feel right, something doesn't feel right, Doc.'

I asked the questions I needed to make the diagnosis and then invited him to go to the examining room. I asked Jonathan to take off his clothes from the waist up and to lie down on the couch.

He started to cough, a very unique cough.

I waited respectfully, at a distance, and a safe angle away from potentially infected droplets, as I always do. I then approached him with the stethoscope fitted in my ears, sphygmomanometer in my right hand ready to be put around the arm of the patient.

Jonathan was silent, looking in the opposite direction. He was suffering, I could feel it. I started my examination and observed in silence. There were large, round, deep purple patches on his skin, like large bruises. These were not bruising. I recognised in an instant the lesions I'd seen more than twenty years ago on a patient dying from AIDS in the Parisian hospital. These round, deep purple skin lesions were due to a rare condition called Kaposi's sarcoma. I remembered it well now. These lesions were pathognomonic, they were specifically and uniquely indicative of AIDS.

I completed the physical examination, kept at a safe distance to avoid droplets from the cough, while Jonathan intuitively kept facing the opposite way. I then kindly asked the sick man to get dressed and to join me in the office.

'Jonathan, you need to be admitted to a specialist ward. Let me call the hospital.'

'I know, thanks, Doc.' The man remained silent in between a few more coughing fits while I dialled the hospital. I was put through to the specialist service and thankfully was soon talking to the consultant in charge!

'Good afternoon, thank you for taking my call. I have with me a male patient of thirty-five years of age, he is presenting with a cough of more than five months along with Kaposi's sarcoma skin lesions all over the torso. Can you arrange his transport?'

'Yes, of course.'

'Please send them directly.'

Ten minutes later, Jonathan was gone.

I went immediately to talk to the receptionist. And, to my surprise, she already knew! Even before I had time to explain, the tiny and tidy receptionist said,

'I know, Dr. Elpis. The man has TB, this cough, poor guy. Do not worry, Doctor, he did not stay long in the waiting room, and no one was even there. When I saw the man and heard his cough, I knew and, in fact, I was about to call and alert you, but you saw him without any wait.'

The woman was a retired nurse, who has worked in both Saint Bartholomew and Middlesex hospitals between the sixties and eighties. In those times, she was working hard under the scrutiny of a matron educated according to Florence Nightingale's precepts. She saw a few cases of TB. She knew that Jonathan had TB just by the sound of it.

Together, we got on with our long-learned duties, as we had in the past. We both cleaned everything, spraying disinfectant everywhere without thinking, automatically doing what we had been taught to do so long ago. I did not wear my white hospital coat, and the receptionist did not wear her blue uniform with apron, the blue Petersham belt with the silver buckle, and her plain cap from the seventies' Middlesex hospital. However, we did all the things we had learned to do.

And the day went on. I called David. He was grateful Jonathan had finally got access to modern medical treatment. And life went on.

Jonathan stayed at the hospital and David visited him, as permitted.

However, and sadly, the young man died just a few weeks later. The AIDS and TB had gone too far already. Both conditions had already damaged the lungs, the blood cells, the liver. The human body was already losing the battle against germs and the virus. It was too late for any rescue, no matter how sophisticated it could have been. The medical treatment did not work and Jonathan, the young man with woolly hair, died at the age of thirty-five in a hospital of the twenty-first century.

David was in despair and felt hopeless. He came to see me, wept, and told me how the whole story saddened him.

'There was no family around, no loved ones. I was the only person who went to see him. I could not approach him though. I was just waving behind the window and left when I could perceive a sort of reply from him.'

I listened kindly but with some anger and sadness in my heart. I could not help but feel angry. Why did nobody spot the AIDS or TB before? Jonathan attended his GP practice on several occasions, many certificates were filled in, many prescriptions were written. He even went to the local hospital when he couldn't cope with the sleepless nights, fatigue and aches all over his body.

His symptoms were easy to spot by a trained doctor who pays attention to details, has a sense of care and a systematic approach to diagnosing infectious disease. In the 5th century BC, Hippocrates and his colleagues were excellent at picking up on TB, why could doctors of the twenty-first century not be?

My anger toward misdiagnosis calmed down though, and days went on, one after another.

A few years later, I received by email an invitation to a conference at the Royal Society of Medicine with the impressive and interesting title: *Royal Society of Medicine TB Day conference 2019: Recent progress and the path towards elimination*. I remembered Jonathan's sad case and decided to go.

On the day of the conference, I was sitting comfortably in a luxurious green armchair in the high-tech Max Rayne Auditorium of the Royal Society of Medicine. We were all awaiting the first speaker. I read the document I had been given. The attendance list was at the back. Mostly nurses but also experts in public health and some hospital physicians were attending. No GP names to be seen, only I, a private GP from Harley Street. I felt different and alone!

The meeting started. Six speakers, one after another, presented recent data, work and research. A professor from Denmark presented his work on his country and Indonesia, with a full chapter on a brand-new, modern, close to nature aseptic sanatorium. Then, the UK Head of Public Health showed the benefits of the recent countrywide measures, such as track, tracing and detection prior to immigration. She also made a point of the persistence of delayed diagnoses. She told us that on average, it takes four months of visiting doctors to be finally diagnosed with TB, and that this delay in diagnosis had not been altered or improved with the new countrywide measures. I listened and understood: Jonathan' s case was not unusual after all.

Then, Professor K talked about the UK treatment of multidrug-resistant TB, the protocols, the necessary isolation of these patients for several months and the difficulties in treating them, with old-fashioned treatments with so many side effects.

He then showed a photograph of the dedicated hospital room in his hospital for these patients. The audience was shocked, and many questions came forth. How on earth could we not be like our colleagues in Denmark? Why could we not have a purpose-built sanatorium with large windows, open to nature, a comfortable room with space, a TV set, and colours to appease the mind of these unfortunate people? How could someone stay isolated in a small hospital room without access to the outside world even by means of a TV for months? Could you? I could not.

The audience was obviously sad and despairing. Why were we tolerating such predicaments in our profession? We were all sitting in the high-tech Max Rayne auditorium, but we were at a loss. I felt sorry for Professor K who, despite the odds, obviously cared for his patients while doing his utmost for the community. The man would later tell me in confidence,

'Compassion, that is what I need the most in my job.'

Following the conference, I felt sad and not optimistic at all. I came back home, sweet home, and sat in my armchair in silence. I decided at once to let it go in favour of daydreaming, which should soothe my nerves. As easily as I can be instantly transported back to my childhood through a piece of art, I can also decide to welcome my forefather for a moment of serenity in the face of hardship. That generally helps me to face the confusions of this world.

Tonight, no reading. Curled in my preferred position, the goose down pillow tucked under my head, feet intertwined, hands between thighs feeling the warmth, three deep breaths, I got set for my imagination to run free, for my daydreaming.

Hippocrates and I are in the sitting room, him on the sofa, me on the opposite armchair.

I say, 'Hippocrates, you understand now that British people are not the most remote of Earth's people.'

'My dear friend from the future, I do understand. Earth is round, and distance is relative. My dear sister in the profession, we have had a big day. I am so exhausted by all these novelties and this new medical understanding. We should now relax and think.'

'Hippocrates, I am glad you understand the value of my telepathic experience at the Royal Academy. You know so much, Hippocrates. You know already what neuroscientists of today are uncovering, that imagination is so important to healthy human function.'

'This is true; however, we did not understand the connections of diseases with live matters that you call germs, viruses or parasites, or the idea of contagiousness. Do tell me, Elpis. I comprehend that your predecessors have scientifically demonstrated that miasma does not exist. According to your current knowledge, diseases, the ones you call infectious diseases, are transmitted by a live matter you call a germ, a virus or a parasite ...

I also comprehend the derived notion of communicable disease and the need to sometimes not follow the oath. I understand doctors notify cases to authorities for the sole purpose of protecting the community by limiting the communicable disease in time and place, and in doing so preventing epidemics. However, is that ethical?

I feel at a loss seeing some patients affected by Tuberculosis B locked down for months in a bare hospital room without any freedom or access to friendship, love, art, music or even nature!'

'Dear Hippocrates, I am also saddened by the predicament of these patients. It is simply inhuman. NHS is still not addressing the situation. Although the medication is free in the country, the access to and completion of the treatment, which can take months, is impaired by the inexistence of a dedicated sanatorium, the lack of community solidarity and of cohesion between the NHS, social services and charities.'

At the time sanatoriums existed, not long ago, diagnosis was made swiftly, and many patients were cured with dignity and by well-trained staff and doctors.

With the disappearance of TB as a major public health issue, these institutions just closed and medical knowledge nearly disappeared. As for today, the disease is still in the background for a few, and resistance of the germ is problematic.

Hippocrates, other countries around the world have built sanatoriums of the twenty-first century for people affected by the disease and in need of isolation for proper treatment. People can rest and recuperate in safety and dignity in these places. In Denmark for example, doctors can treat their patients in a dedicated sanatorium where patients have access to nature, art and comfort.'

'My dear Elpis, your world can be so rough, I cannot help but think with tears of Jonathan and his last hours in this tiny room, all alone, far from nature and humanity. It seems that despite many new scientific discoveries and concepts, the rational world of yours can allow neglect and inhuman treatment when simple willpower and will to do good could resolve it all.

Your world is so unkind, my dear Elpis.'

I listened, despondent, but could not talk in return.

In a graceful gesture, Hippocrates takes his special lyre, the kithara.

'My kind Elpis, let's play music, we both need to soothe our hearts. Let's get some serenity in the face of your world and its contradictions.'"

Silence settled in The Mirage. After a few minutes, Melo kindly murmured,

"Thank you, Doctor. Another instructive daydream. I feel saddened though by Jonathan's story, so unfair."

Elpis did not respond, but nodded, holding her hood on both sides. This was a nod as good as a wink. Melo kept silent, smiled at the doctor while imagining the *Hakushiko Noh* mask underneath the hood. She then said,

"Doctor, I am fascinated by the nearly instant diagnosis you made, just by observing Jonathan's skin."

"A lot has to do with experience, I guess. I have seen so much skin in my life. Looking at you, Melo, I can tell that you are healthy, that you have sufficient outdoor activities, you eat your five portions of fruit and vegetables, and that you are of Celtic background."

"Dr. Elpis, I am not so sure of that. I love eating Mars bars, hamburgers and carrot cakes. Furthermore, I have no Celtic background at all. We have been Anglo-Saxon for many generations."

The doctor did not reply and got back to her quiet, static posture, both hands on the wooden tabletop, quietly joined together as if in prayer.

"Good story, Doctor." Melo packed the black Moleskine notebook along with the pen box. She was ready to go.

"Bye Doctor, bye Mia."

While I continue to keep this oath unviolated, may it be granted to me to enjoy life and the practice of the art, respected by all men, in all times!

HIPPOCRATES

Saturday Eleven

Melo talked to her father about Celtic genes. The man said, without hesitation, "We are Anglo-Saxons and have been so for many generations. Dr. Elpis is wrong."

Melo did not discuss it further. She sensed the subject was upsetting in some way. And anyway, Melo was more interested in talking to Brian. She liked his view on life. Brian was studying Geopolitics, Resources and Territory at Kings College London. He liked talking about urbanism and shared his view on coworking environments. They talked and talk. He then told her about the ancient Celtic beliefs and rituals related to agriculture, and before she left, he invited her to join him for Halloween. She accepted.

On the eleventh Saturday, Melo arrived at The Mirage at 6.56 am and parked her beloved cherry-red bicycle with Mia at the door, waiting for her.

"Hi, good morning. Let me take your overcoat, you're soaked!"

"Oh, thank you, Mia. The rain has not stopped since I left Richmond. I feel so good though. And I am on time! I was really worried I may not make it."

"Come through. Matcha tea?"

"And a carrot cake too please, this ride has built my appetite. I feel I could eat like an ogre. Oh, by the way, Brian and I went up Primrose Hill last night. It was cathartic, it was like we both connected with the spiritual moon."

"What? I'll bring your tea and the cake."

Mia went off with the wet raincoat and repeated in her mind with a little smile, 'Cathartic', whatever that is, on Primrose Hill, a spiritual moon? The girl is a real nerd. Brian? Brian. Briiiiian, of course, I knew it.

Melo walked through The Mirage and smiled at the sight of the familiar hooded figure in the dim light.

"Good morning, Melo. Take this towel, you shouldn't stay like that, your legs are all wet."

"Oh thank you, Doctor. Not to worry, I am going to change anyway. I brought some dry clothes with me."

Melo dried her long legs and then went downstairs. In a few minutes, she was back, her long curls freed and bouncing.

"I like your T-shirt. It's terrific, is it from Drop Dead?"

"Yes, Drop Dead is my favourite British fashion brand. I'm happy you know it."

"It is a killer if I may say so, just terrific. It is so pretty, the wide-eyed little angel with wings, and her trainers with bloodstains, so cool, so you, Melo!"

"Thank you. It's funny you say that. I feel that way. You know, I identify myself with the angel on my T-shirt. My generation that I call the digital natives is simply displacing the notion of fame and ego within the variables of reality. This is my anthropologist's view, I guess. Virtual fame can be for one day and for anyone, in the virtual or real world, or both, and that is cool. Also, what you call 'ego' can be for us a manga, or a character created from scratch on the web or playing games, connecting in social media, or even wearing meaningful clothes."

Melo thought of Brian and reflected. She did not understand or even know him yet, let alone his ego, but she knew he was real and connected to her, to her very being.

Elpis then said, "Interesting, Melo. I also think that the very meaning of both fame and ego are changing in a big way. It is like ego can be augmented by the smartphone and the immediate access to a virtual world. Ego can also get closer to our DNA. The space-time dimension of our very being is nowadays transforming all the time, at high speed, sometimes getting smaller, sometimes bigger, sometimes inward, and other times outward. It is like the world we perceive has become elastic, constantly changeable, as if pulsating.

And we humans should be in permanent resonance in this new non-linear world."

"This is becoming complicated, Doctor. Let us come back round to you. Are you a famous doctor?"

"I am not, Melo, I told you at the beginning. I am just a messenger."

"A messenger for a famous Harley Street doctor?"

"No Melo, I am the messenger of the art of medicine.

I am averse to self-promotion. A good friend of mine said that I was a doctor without ego. I am an inconsequential being. And yet, I have not ceased to examine who I am with the objective of always being a better person."

The doctor added, "Are you warm now? Is the carrot cake nice?"

"Yummy, yummy." Melo chewed a tiny piece of the cake, swallowed, and said, "I have a boyfriend. He is called Brian. He's so cool."

The doctor pulled down the right side of her hood. Melo smiled at the wink. The doctor then sat back, entwined her fingers, only the kiss of death ring today, wrists resting on the table. Melo stared and imagined the *Hakushiko* mask with its peaceful smile.

She took another miniature piece of cake, then one of her three pens from the box, and waited.

"I am not a famous doctor, I have never been listed in Tatler, thankfully. I am an independent doctor, judged by others for my actions and not for who I am. Being independent has helped me to follow the ancient and universal wisdom, but it was my long carrier and experience which has allowed me to tell you, the anthropologist, my stories, and I must say that you have so far succeeded in capturing the very essence of what I've said. I thank you for that.

To illustrate the words, 'While I continue to keep this oath unviolated, may it be granted to me to enjoy life and the practice of the art, respected by all men, in all times!', I propose to tell you about the first ever rock concert I went to.

It was in 2017. I went incognito and on my own to see Melvin's gig in Camden, Koko Theatre."

"Melvin's! A great band, I did not know they'd been in London.

Sorry, Doctor, do carry on."

"I travelled by tube. It was late autumn and, by 6 pm, it was already dark. Near Warren Street tube station, a group of Romanian homeless people were gathered, all sitting on the pavement. I reckoned that they had been gathering near the station for more than two years at least.

I observed and concluded it was the end of their day's begging. These people were behaving like their counterparts with homes and jobs who meet in a pub at the end of a working day. Most were laughing, smiling to each other, talking together, one or two were clearly dating, there was some 'Love Com' energy there. Others were huddled together, staring at a mobile phone screen, the usual behaviour following a day of work in London."

"Doctor, you could be an anthropologist too," Melo murmured, still writing.

"Oyster card out of my pocket a few seconds before the arrival at the underground gates, a touch of the contactless card to the yellow reader, gate opening. I was now walking down the escalator. I felt good that day. I had the intense feeling of being part of the city I love so much. I had that *omoiyari* feeling too, I was conscientiously considerate to my fellow Londoners."

The doctor carried on. "On my feet, my creeper boots, the platforms I'd bought for the concert."

"Doctor, I have to say, these shoes suit you very well indeed."

"Thank you. Did you know that since the fifties in Manchester, the shoes have remained the same? I always wanted to get some. I love the design, with the range of three D-ring laces, and its signature lace apron. The construction on a walled round-toe is the most adapted to my ageing feet, which need comfort. You will know one day."

Melo thought of her mother's feet.

"So, let's come back to that day I went to Koko. It was cold, 5 degrees Celsius according to my iPhone.

On arrival, I went downstairs to be close to the musicians. The place was already packed.

I observed and rapidly felt overwhelmed by the humanity of it all. Music was the drug.

I remember Dale Crover settled in front of his drums, then Steve McDonald, Jeff Pinkus, and King Buzzo with his mighty hair. He was wearing a terrific black kaftan with one large satanic eye on the front.

The music started. In an instant, I got into it. These guys know what they are doing, they really do! The whole audience stood, listened, and enjoyed with mind and body and as one the sounds and melodies. The brain and primary auditory cortex were stimulated simultaneously. The chaotic brain was functioning at its best for most of us.

'Don't forget to breathe!' Buzzo was shouting to us all.

Despite my underground platform shoes, most people were taller than me. However, and amazingly, I could sense a tiny clearing around me. The group moved slightly to allow *la petite dame* to see, and when the music became releasing and cathartic, there was another palpable concerted movement to create a barrage, to prevent the tiny woman with creeper boots being hurt. I was pushed away from the mosh pit. The headbangers were already in a trance, with sudden waves of movement and headbanging.

Nobody got hurt despite the craziness of the whole situation, the group was one and protective of the weaker.

I observed with contentment the humanity of it all, its unalterable group attitude and defence of the weaker: me, the tiny human being with creeper boots.

I felt safe and so good. I sensed the music inside and outside my body; I felt part of something grand. Pure joy was flooding out of me. I felt the catharsis of the moment and I was at peace and content. Much better than meditation, I can tell you!

'Don't forget to breathe,' Buzzo, Steve Shane Mac Donald and Jeff Pinkus were all singing in concert. The music was perfectly played.

I breathed in and out, in and out, my head banging rhythmically. Music passed through the skilled fingers of the musicians to link the unconscious to the conscious and spread through the air, to connect all the brains and bodies around them.

It was a new reality to my world!

Melo, I have often been fascinated and taken aback by the irreducible part of a patient unravelling in front of me, a doctor. In Koko, for the first time in my life, I saw and felt the irreducible part of a human group.

I thought and pondered. Humanity is strong when the group spirit is alive! It was a naïve thought, but it gave me hope.

The moment at Koko stayed in my mind for several weeks though. The music did not become an earworm or a musical obsession, but this group experience remained in my mind for a long time.

Thereafter, life went on as usual. In the news, a lot was happening. I remember well two pieces of news.

A lost portrait of the young Charles Dickens was found in a South African market, covered in mould next to a metal lobster! It was a gouache and watercolour, only 14 cm, from Margaret Gillies. Charles Dickens appeared as a young ephebe with big eyes, clean-shaven, with long wavy hair, in contrast to the portraits of the older Dickens we have all become accustomed to. According to the newspaper, Dickens in the portrait was in his early thirties. Older people have all been young once! However, the soul does not age. I wanted to understand this very idea. I carefully compared the eyes of this portrait with William Powell Frith's one, when Dickens was much older. The gaze, *le regard*, the mirror of the soul was identical! Incredible, no? the gaze was identical, time had not affected it in any way. I was convinced. The soul is timeless."

"Interesting, Doctor. My grandmother's eyes are so crystal clear you know, I have always been amazed by them. I will look at old photos tonight for comparison."

Elpis did not reply and stayed silent for a few seconds. Melo broke the silence and said:

"Doctor, what about the other fascinating news of that week?"

"Tarita Alarcón Rapu, the governor of Easter Island, met with the British Museum director, wearing her crown made of sacred white feathers. Her people wanted Hoa Hakananai'a back. She claimed

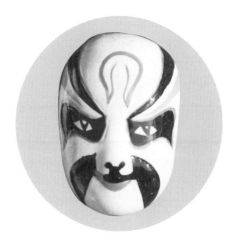

that it was the very soul of her nation. She did not obtain what she wanted, yet this was the opening of positive negotiations between the two countries.

Other and not less important news got announced or published that week.

Donald Trump was tweeting in the background! Political correctness seemed at a loss with this new political communication route. And Brexit was still tottering along! French civil unrest was reported too. The activists were named the Yellow Vests. They came from nowhere, a surprise to all. These people were shouting to be heard, to be respected, and were gathering together on roundabouts, blocking the roads and demonstrating week after week in several French cities, with even guerrilla scenes on Champs-Élysées avenue.

And the most destructive and deadly wildfire was growing in California and had been since mid-July!

That week, Sir David Attenborough was preparing his speech to the United Nation climate change summit in Poland. 'The collapse of civilisation and of the natural world is on the horizon,' he will say."

Melo stopped writing, gazed at the doctor and said, "My mother keeps talking about climate change."

"So let's get back to my week.

That week, something else, amazing news caught my attention. Some scientists had developed a software able to mimic in real-time how the brain naturally activates the spinal cord. We may be able to make a paraplegic walk again by retraining his brain with a computer! The study was named STIMO.

Melo, this is serious and complicated stuff. Are you Ok if I go through it with you today?"

"Of course, Doctor. Anyway, I can check Google later."

"When I started my medical studies in the early eighties, it was thought that once the brain was disconnected from a part of the body, as in paraplegia, there was no possibility of any kind of reconnection. It was thought the neurones could not be repaired. This was later proved to be wrong with the discovery of the brain and neurones' plasticity. A natural occurrence of repair at the brain or neuronal level called neuronal plasticity was in fact possible. And STIMO has proved that the machine can trigger the natural phenomenon of repair and plasticity.

The study was published in *Nature Neuroscience* and became readable that very week on the internet.

STIMO means Stimulation Movement Overground. It is the first human study to confirm the safe feasibility of a closed-loop Epidural Electrical Stimulation, EES, in combination with overground robot-assisted rehabilitation training.

The experiment is complicated and difficult to understand, I know, but let me try to explain the main findings to you in simple words.

So, the researchers have managed to 'wake up' a part of a brain, the part which was disconnected as the result of the paraplegia, and which normally processes proprioception signals coming via the spinal cord from the receptors. Proprioception has been called the sixth sense. It is the sense of the relative position of one's parts of the body and of their strength. Proprioception is necessary for a human being to walk when it is not as essential for an animal. In some ways, proprioception, the sixth sense, makes us human and enables us to dance or to play an instrument, to jump, smile, and so on and so forth."

"Dr. Elpis, how does proprioception work?"

"The brain integrates information from proprioception through the nerves which travel through the spinal cord and which are connected to receptors in the muscles, joints and skin, together with the signals from the vestibular system in the ears. Then, the brain establishes its overall sense of body position, movement and acceleration.

The brains of paraplegics are disconnected from their muscles, joints and skin receptors because of a breakdown of the transmission at spinal cord level. Their brain cannot identify the position, movement and acceleration of the lower limbs. Paraplegics cannot move their legs.

While animals can walk again with simple electrical stimulation of a nerve, human beings need a system replacing proprioception, a system sending complex and variable proprioceptive information to the brain. That is what the computer and the EES system, the Epidural Electrical Stimulation, has been able to achieve.

During the STIMO study, patients recovered voluntary control of leg muscles that had been paralysed for many years. After a few months of training, they were able to control previously paralysed leg muscles even in the absence of electrical stimulation. In other words, their brains had relearned the lost skills and could independently link with the limbs. Proprioception was awakened, but only partly.

According to the YouTube video, the walking of the paraplegic, even if amazing from the scientific and technological point of view, is very awkward and mechanistic, not human enough yet. It is limited in a lot of ways and may not be satisfying for the patient. Proprioception is a very complex human sense, and even if STIMO study results are amazing from a technological point of view, it is still uncertain that the machine will enable paraplegics to fully regain the complexity of their sixth sense. Furthermore, the ethical dilemma surrounding these technologies have not yet been addressed.

'While I continue to keep this oath unviolated, may it be granted to me to enjoy life and the practice of the art, respected by all men, in all times!'

The Hippocratic oath's sentence cannot apply to the STIMO computer, the EES, to neuroscientists or techies either. But one day, I hope, the technology will have passed all the ethical tests and doctors will be confident enough to prescribe the technology and make paraplegics walk again."

Silence settled in The Mirage. Melo thought of Jack, a friend of the family, who has been paraplegic following a road accident. Then the doctor said:

"But for now, my dear Melo, it is time to leave each other. Next Saturday will be our last meeting, which will be a few days before Halloween."

Then, the doctor added, "Let's plan something special, should we? Yes, same time, same place, but with our chosen costumes for Halloween."

"That's grand," replied Melo. "So see you next week."

Melo left without further words. Mia, busy behind the bar, winked at her friend.

Outside The Mirage, Melo's phone bleeped. A message, a waving Yoda sticker and a black witch. Melo smiled and walked on.

Later on that day, Melo looked at the YouTube video of the STIMO study with her parents. Her father thought the paraplegic was walking like a zombie. He then raised the possible dangerous use of such a technology: What if people could not choose using it? What if the NHS took the opportunity of such a technology to stop offering wheelchairs? Her mother added that anyway, the NHS was not offering out free modern and powered wheelchairs, and that the few disabled people one could see were the happy ones who had been helped in other ways. Things were complicated and sad for many, they all thought. To try to get back some optimism, Father and Mother talked about Jack and how he managed to stay positive and strong, despite his injury.

But should I trespass and violate this oath, may the reverse be my lot!

HIPPOCRATES

Saturday Twelve

The Saturday before Halloween was the day of the last meeting with the doctor.

At 6.59 am, Melo entered The Mirage, thinking of herself as her drummer's Igraine: the mother of King Arthur and Morgana.

Was she in love? She did not know. The night before, though, a lot happened. Brian painted a green spot between her eyes, from which he designed and painted a Celtic tree of life. On each side of the branches, on her cheeks, he painted three leafy, white branches. The young man then carefully attached golden sweet chestnut leaves in her hair and whispered in Melo's ears,

"Be my Igraine, beautiful chick."

Melo loved it, it was so cool! And today, she felt as if something subliminal was caressing each of her cells. Melo felt that she was Brian's Igraine, down to her spine. Was that love? Was Brian to become her second half?

Melo chose not to wear the long dress her mother had bought her for last year's Halloween. Mia sent her some drawings of a giant girl with curly red hair and a long, wavy, transparent black dress, walking with a tiny black witch. Melo was inspired and decided to wear metallic pale-gold skinny jeans. Around the waist, the black, see-through chiffon mesh maxi skirt she'd bought last year was waving slightly. Melo loved its long side slits; it gave her a feeling of physical freedom. She felt ephemeral as she walked. The balance of the skirt was just magical, especially with her yellow platform trainers. So cool, so wicked!

Melo arrived at The Mirage. Mia was behind the bar with her phone. She raised her eyes and gazed in admiration at Melo.

"Wow, this is a killer. I like the tree!"

With a big smile, Melo winked to her friend in return and walked to the doctor.

"My dear, you are so beautiful."

Melo could not help but blush. However, she kept her back straight and her shoulders back. She was delighted to be with the doctor on that special day and forgot it was for the last time.

She was surprised though. Elpis did not have a hoodie on. Rather, she was wearing a plain mask. Melo did not think of the absence of *Hakushiko*'s peaceful smile which she had imagined so often before. She was instead interested in the yellow-brown snake with scales edged in white painted on the left side of the mask. The snake's body was crossing half the forehead, with its long, triangular, slender head and round, red pupils just between the doctor's eyes.

Elpis was wearing a black dress with a sweetheart neckline which suited her impeccably.

"The snake is beautiful, Doctor. I suppose it is an Aesculapian one, is that correct?"

"Yes, well spotted. You know your classics, well done! Melo, you are beautiful. I just love the tree of life and the autumn colours on you. The sweet chestnut tree leaves are so cleverly entangled in your golden hair. Only magic or love can do that."

"Thank you, you are beautiful too. And, and … Elpis, I have brought a gift specially for you: a magpie crossbones and pearl chain necklace."

"My dear friend, well chosen! It is beautiful, I love it!"

The two women laughed together. Happiness was in the air.

"My turn, Melo. Here is a gift for you, a kithara, the lyre Hippocrates used to play to his patients. A Greek master luthier has done it specially for you."

"This is just wonderful, thank you so much."

Melo held the instrument with amazement and great respect, touched the wood and the seven strings with emotion. She felt the urge to play and wanted to hold Elpis and kiss her too. She could not though; they were both too studious, too regimented. But maybe not.

Melo just sensed that if she kissed Elpis, her blood would change to honey. Magic was in the air.

However, Melo knew that Dr. Elpis was not a shaman or a witch, or even a messenger. Elpis was a human doctor, loved by the mythical gods, and that her own sense of *omoiyari* was synonymous with the doctor's idea of compassion. Melo thought of one of her father's words: 'posthumanism'. Yes, Elpis was a post-humanist doctor, and Melo liked her very much indeed.

Melo respectfully positioned the kithara by her side and sat down. She took out her Moleskine notebook and a pen from the silver pen box.

"Dear Melo, I really doubt that fame for any doctor should go beyond the number of patients he or she is able to treat. However, I know that damnation of a doctor by a community, a country, or even the entire world is possible and sometimes inevitable. You may remember about Dr. Karl Brandt. I talked to you about him on the third Saturday we met and discussed euthanasia. Karl Brandt was certainly the most disruptive doctor of the twentieth century. His law on euthanasia led to the deaths of so many people. After the war, he was sentenced to death at the Doctors' trial by a US military tribunal, and later hanged on the 2nd of June 1948.

Unfortunately, the current quest for artificial intelligence in health-care is pushing some of my colleagues to violate the oath once again and to take risks for the profession at their own expense.

The development of Babylon Healthcare is one example of what is happening right now.

Let me tell you the truth.

Babylon Healthcare is developing an Algorithm for medical diagnosis. It is a British company named after a bogus historical fact with a chimeric mission, nothing less. Its founders claim that 2500 years ago, the Babylonians were the healthiest people in the world because they were sharing, on the marketplace, ideas and knowledge about minor ailments and traditional remedies. This statement, to be read by all on the web, is one example of what the post-truth era of twenty-first century pseudoscience can produce: a bogus historical and pseudoscientific statement. It is simply wrong.

First, the statement creates ambiguity between community health and medicine. Second, it confuses minor ailments and diseases, and lastly, it is based on a false historical fact. Greeks, probably North American Indians, and others were at that time as healthy as the Babylonians.

The truth, as you now know, is that scientific medicine was created 2500 years ago by Hippocrates and his school of Kos. They may have cooperated with Babylonian doctors, but not on the marketplaces! Hippocrates died at the tender age of ninety, some say eighty-three, but even still, he was healthy and had never been part of a crowded marketplace. He did not share opinions with commoners. Hippocrates disregarded opinions and divine beliefs. He was the founder and protector of scientific medicine, based on empiricism and not opinions or beliefs. He doctored according to his principles, visiting patients in their homes, always respecting their privacy, and was venerated as one of the best physicians by other scientists of his time.

Furthermore, community health, what Babylon Healthcare is referring to, has nothing to do with the resolution of minor ailments or even medicine! This is so stupid. What does make a healthy community is a healthy diet in a healthy societal and natural environment, along with sanitation. Nothing more, nothing less. Sanitation, healthy environment and diet.

Medicine or healthcare, even free for all, does not alone translate to an improvement in the health of a nation. We should all know this.

However, Babylon Healthcare has a mission. It is to bring healthcare to all humanity, a utopic and demagogic dream in my view. However, the company is supported by many and is working hard at it. Global investors have joined and are waiting for results. An algorithm is developed day by day, thanks to the clever machine-learning system linked to a chatbot. Patients can call and chat to a doctor anytime of the day or night. Then dutifully, patients fill in a satisfaction questionnaire and get a prescription as a reward. That sounds great to many, but not to me, Melo. Not to me. And, in the background, medical data is collected every night and day to develop the machine learning system and its algorithm.

Common sense, compassion and empathy are all out of the artificial intelligence equation, of course. A machine cannot have common sense, let alone compassion or even empathy.

Human doctors, medicine, and its Hippocratic principles seem to be out of the equation too, from conception to development.

Not long ago, the company staged an experiment, pitting its algorithm against trainee doctors in a diagnostic test, and then claimed that the machine proved superior. The trainees were not named and the personal effect of their bad results against the machine were not considered at all.

The trainees, the doctors-to-be who lost in front of the machine stayed unnamed and were just forgotten. However, the press and Forbes Magazine ran a piece under the headline *AI just beat human doctors on a medical exam*, and the medical director of the company got nominated the most influential GP in the world.

That is what happened.

And the algorithm is developing further and further. With its current exponential development, it is likely we shall have soon an algorithm replacing a GP. And when this happens, this doctor, the most influential GP glorified by Forbes, could become the most disruptive medical doctor of the twenty-first century.

Dear Melo, I'm annoyed, and I have been so since that Babylon's experiment. I am infuriated that no one is questioning what is happening with artificial intelligence in healthcare.

Let's face it, Babylon is developing a system with a false vision and without thinking of the potential future consequences. It is developing a system to match the average human intelligence, in total denial of compassion or common sense but also in denial of the clinicians, the doctors directly involved in the treatment of the patient.

Even if the machine is using the most advanced self-learning system with convolutional networks, even if it is learning fast with the availability of the data people produce daily, on a twenty-four-hour basis, even if the system will improve as a result, there is something fundamentally wrong here.

What about care, common sense, compassion, trust and responsibility? What about techies, pseudoscientists and experts using false historical statements dreaming of a chimeric world? What about a doctor recognised as the most influential in a society because of his business acumen and demagogic vision, but not for his medical care or respect of the oath?

This seems evil to me!

And furthermore, what about bias in the conception of the machine and the probable human's profiling?

This seems evil to me too!"

Melo interrupted, "Profiling is anthropologically damaging and dangerous, but nobody cares."

"Babylon Healthcare is probably the most unwise and potentially dangerous healthcare adventure there is, to my mind, but it is not the only one. Entrepreneurs, techies, politicians, experts, pharmaceutical industries, global charities, doctors all around the world are joining the movement.

The Gates Foundation has been running a new program called CEPI, the coalition for Epidemic Preparedness Innovations with the dream of vaccinating anybody on Earth. Google is running a programme called Verily with the mission of mapping human health. Facebook has moved into data analytics and healthcare advertising. IBM's Watson programme, with its natural language, hypothesis generation and evidence-based learning capabilities is now involved in management decisions about lung cancer treatment in the USA. Its capabilities are currently being investigated in terms of contributing to human doctors' clinical decisions. Apple has developed its new Apple Watch Series 4, with a proactive health monitor and an integrated ECG! In London, biotech companies have been popping up out of nowhere. New companies and research units have been created from scratch and promote enhancements in prevention, diagnostics and therapies, you name it.

I am saddened and dismayed by the whole thing. Doctors have already lost their powerful position regarding medical knowledge due to the development of the internet, and may soon lose control of prescription, diagnosis, prognosis and even treating epidemics. Doctors may simply disappear.

Melo, this is the reason I have decided to talk to you. For years, I have been reading about digital disruption. I tried to keep open mind and to welcome the inevitable technological transformation of my profession. However, the neglect of the industry for ethical fundamentals, the disconnection between the techies' dreams and the people, the greed all of these upset me on and on. I kept thinking technology was not dangerous, but what about the large sum of money invested in it? What's it for? And then, I realised that more than greed, the transhumanism ideology was at stake, and that political leaders did not see through it. Transhumanism was undermining the humanity of it all.

Transhumanists are atheists who believe that technology shall increase human capacities, that AI shall become cleverer than all of us, and that control but also eternity could be granted to some.

One night, the night of my mother's twenty-sixth death anniversary, I had a nightmare which will stay engraved in my memory forever.

I was lying down, without any cloth, on a medical couch similar to the one used during my radiotherapy sessions.

I felt a dense 37 degree Celsius flow dripping down my side, a river of blood. It was warm, sticky, thick and muddy. I was bleeding.

Adult conjoined female twins with enlarged, bright red lips were standing on my left side. I was looking at them while trying to touch the bleeding part of my body. However, something was preventing me from doing so. I could not move my hand. There was like something else preventing me from moving or even shouting. The obscene scene was silent. I was horrified but could not scream.

I gazed at the twins, who both had the exact same forced and empathetic smile deformed by Botox. Then, they moved close to me and, in one joint movement, approached silently and shaped their bright red lips ready to kiss. I could not move, I could not shout, no sound was coming out of my mouth. It was just horrendous. But then, I felt a sinking ache inside my bleeding breast. I could not move my body away from the lips but managed to turn my head toward the side of the pain.

And what I saw was even scarier. Ray Kurzweil, the famous advocate of transhumanism. In my dream, it was him. The transhumanist I only met on the web, was popping vitamin capsules, one by one, into my mutilated breast.

It was awful, the pain was just unbearable.

I gazed at him, then at the conjoined women, then at him. The man kept popping the capsules in, brutally, and yet with an empathetic smile on his face. I could move my head, but my body was paralysed. It was horrendous.

My attackers all had a letter tattooed in red on their foreheads, a Q or a C. Kurzweil had a Q. It was awful. He kept popping his capsules in, one by one, the Q letter moving, even pulsating on his sweaty skin. My heart was beating fast, I was screaming inside, but still no noise managed to escape from my tortured body. I could not move, my breast was painful, the ache was throbbing. I felt as though my breast was going to explode with all of Kurzweil's red, blue, white and green pills.

But then the moist, cherry-red lips of the women touched my body when Ray whispered in my ear, 'You need help, Doctor, you need help'.

That is when I woke up all sweaty with massive palpitations. I touched my scar. It was bleeding and in pain.

I could not go back to sleep, got up and changed the dressing of my breast. While getting ready for work, I kept thinking of that dream. I felt that I was like Prometheus condemned by the gods to suffer eternally. And then, I realised the truth. I was a Homo Sacer, a human being who cannot be sacrificed to the gods, but who can be killed by the system and the transhumanist techies. I was stuck. As always, I went back to my daily reality and got ready for the day.

I left home though, with the vivid memory of the dream and my acceptance of my condition of Homo Sacer. My death will join the statistics and be transformed into a well-classified number.

I carried on and walked up Marylebone High Street, trying to focus my mind on something else. A boy and his sister were both walking the other way, white Apple earphones between them, connecting a smartphone to the boy's left ear and his sister's right one. He with a cap, very slim, a checked jacket, jeans and blue Converse trainers, a star on the side of each shoe. She, older and taller than him, with long straight hair. A teenager already, simple blue jacket, jeans, and pink Converse Taylor shoes. Christmas lights were shining above our heads, illuminated interweaving stars mirroring the shoes of brother and sister. I was now walking along Weymouth Street, BT Tower on the horizon, its top hidden in the mist of the London sky, with one plane crossing over. It was beautiful.

When I arrived at my office, I passed two builders looking at a mobile phone and laughing in concert at the tiny screen. I passed the two men with a smile and a feeling of contentment in the face of human joy.

I took off my coat, sat at my desk and logged on. I found the computer slow to wake up. While waiting, I intertwined my fingers to rest my hands on my desk, closed my eyes. I made a decision.

From now on and until I die, I will connect with the future. I will tell the truth, carry the message of the oath and help in a very humble way the destruction of the transhumanism ideology. It was time to draw the moral boundary between humanity and the machine.

A long time before, I lost trust in all these psychologists and experts who classify us and believe they can tell people how to live but do not do anything about it. But on that day, I lost trust in political leaders and their ability to protect our humanity."

Melo stopped writing, listened actively, and gazed at the Asclepius snake. She said, "I have grown up with the idea that I did not have empathy, that was so wrong."

"My dear friend, you have got more than empathy, your awareness of *omoiyari* is quite special for a western girl. You are growing, with an already high capability to listen, and this is quite special. I do know that."

Melo stopped writing, raised and turned her head. As if by magic, Mia was sitting by her side, wearing a witch hat. She winked at Melo, who smiled in response, holding back a laugh, and then went back to her writing.

Elpis looked intensely and with admiration the two friends. They were young, connected and full of joy. Silence settled for a few seconds. Then, she said:

"Humanity and its landscape are both colliding with the tech scape. Human beings are in between, but this transformation must happen.

I imagine the outline of a new world, a world of a generation fully aware of the dangers menacing its very existence but equipped to face the challenge. When transhumanism will have been defeated, and when techies, experts and psychologists will have all been told to limit their work to what they know to do and in respect of a clear code of ethics, this new world shall emerge with courageous and independent people back in charge. Empathy shall be augmented with courage, ethics, compassion and *omoiyari*.

The digital native generation, yours, shall rise to regroup and adapt to both environmental and digital changes.

Dear Melo and Mia, your generation will save the planet, and mine has a duty to help. Humanity shall survive and will adapt, as it has always done."

Mia applauded. Melo joined her forever friend and eagerly clapped her hands.

She then said, "Doctor, is that the finale? I want to know more. I have already learned so much from the story of your mother, Kevin, Jonathan, Freddy Mercury, Camille Claudel and others. We have shared a glimpse of their respective lives, yet all of the stories have opened my mind on humanity and medicine. I want to also hear more about genetics and STIMO studies and the like."

"Melo, I am happy to keep telling you about medicine. I also would like you to understand that beyond medicine, one individual story is like the drop of water of the parable by Sadi of Shiraz. Your memory is acting as the oyster and I can guarantee that at one point of time in your life, the recollection of one of the stories I told you will help and shine like the kingly pearl the drop of water became.

I want to keep telling you stories. This is my mission. Let us put some dates in our respective diaries, shall we? I propose the twelve consecutive Saturdays from the 2nd of January 2021."

Melo took her special five-year diary, ticked the dates, and said:

"We will need to talk again about artificial intelligence."

"I agree. I also want to speak about genetics."

"Yes, we will. And about exoskeletons at the Tokyo Olympic Games too!"

"My father is going to the Olympics."

"And I am going too. But for the time being, let us get ready for Halloween."

Melo carefully enveloped her kithara in a green Daunt Books bag. She turned to Mia, gazed at her friend, tears gathering in her eyes. Melo gave Mia a box wrapped in gold paper with colourful skulls drawn on it.

"What is it?" asked Mia, while opening the box and taking care not to damage the paper.

"It is a light box to illuminate and transfer your drawings."

"Smashing!" Mia walked the dimly lit passage to the bar. She came back holding three carrot cakes in a square box and a green container of ceremonial matcha tea powder.

They both kissed goodbye, holding back their tears.

And with Brian's words of love and the intimate belief in Mia's timeless friendship, our heroine left The Mirage and Soho to walk tall into the future and her destiny.

Dear readers from the future, you are the only ones who know what will be. However, and for now, let me tell you.

The doctor shall

Connect with her fellow humans till the end,

Develop her carbon-free intelligence

And

Live her independence and freedom.

The doctor hopes

Her grandchildren to see and hear the turtle dove.

The doctor does not want to die yet,
she will probably never want to.

She wants life to stay on Earth, and human intelligence
to resonate with the blue planet.

The doctor shall

Keep smiling till the end.

And

One day

With grey hair and wrinkles around eyes and lips

Her carbon-free intelligence still enquiring and observing,

The doctor shall

Transfer her knowledge and skills,

Along with the love of humanity and reverence
for Hippocrates

The doctor shall connect till the end

In the renewed and pulsating spacetime reality of London.

Epilogue

31 October 2018, 12.12pm

I am dreaming.

I am lying down in the foetal position. I feel warm, my loving drummer's precious semen between my thighs. I am sleeping, yet enjoy the rhythmic feeling, like cuddling. I feel a warm fat blobby thing on my back, Mocha Dick, the whale of the Thames. The front of my body is bathed within a warm liquid, caressing my skin, going in and out of my ears, nose and lips. My drummer-boy's music in my ears, bump, bump, bump. I love his rapid tempo. The cadence is unique; it mimics the heartbeat. No, it is my drummer's heartbeat, and it is close to me. I am surrounded by it. Bump, bump, bump, my drummer is not here though. I am alone and sleeping. I am dreaming. Bump, bump, bump. It is someone's heart beating, bump, bump, bump. The green man's heart? No, it is the green world's mother, her heart beating, bump, bump, bump. 70 beats per minute, 120, 130 beats per minutes. I am half-asleep, yet enjoy the rhythmic feeling, like cuddling.

I am dreaming. I am not moving. The pulsing lub and dub accelerates. Something is pushing me, a thing all around me. I am in a smooth and warm envelope, and it is now contracting all around me, pushing my head out. I am pushed rhythmically. I do not move, I just let myself go. I am pushed further; my head is now expelled from the closed envelope in a smooth and warm tight passage. I am gently pushed again, I move further up the warm tight channel-like passage, my neck, torso and tummy are all passing through, all gently, all smoothly.

I am dreaming. My head now leaves the organic, warm, tight passage, to be surrounded by earth. Autumn soil is around me, I am pushed further, then my neck and my torso were both out of the passage in the soil, like the tree's roots, the mycorrhizal network and the worms all around me. The forces of the green world's mother are still at work: I am pushed further up.

I am expelled, all my body is now out of the underworld. I have emerged, and in one movement, I unfold my body to stand upright and proud.

One howl, my lungs open, filling with air. I breathe. The blood circulation switches from the heart through the semilunar valves to the arteries then to the veins, the lungs and then back to the heart. My blood is flowing in one direction, the flow of human life.

I am alive, I am reborn.

I stand at the top of Primrose Hill. I see many people around. At the top, Hippocrates is sitting at Guinevere's round table, along with Elpis, Machaon, Podalirius, Polybius, Professor K, Plato, Aristotle, Diogenes of Sinope, Pythagoras, Euclid, and Ptolemy. A boy with my green bicycle helmet is sitting between Hippocrates and Elpis. On the side of the round table, Pandora's Box is fully open, with the words TB, AIDS, mosquitoes, cancer cells, plastic particles, virus, trolls, C and Q letters dotted around, Asperger, and other indeterminate evils turning and turning above, along with drones of all kinds.

I am not scared, not at all. I stand with a feeling of peace in my core and an earthly nature of being, smelling earth and moss. I observe the world around me with my piercing green eyes. I do not know who I am, I do not know who I have become.

Everyone is here. Many children and elderly people are celebrating. I can see Jason and the Argonauts, Jonathan, Terentius neo, husband and wife, Plato, Kevin with his soft, coiled platinum wire in his brain. I recognise, further down, Camille Claudel holding Rodin's bust like a baby, Freddy Mercury and Scaramouche. On the other side, Jesus Christ is walking with Elpis' mother and the virgin from Michelangelo's Pietà, along with Grandma.

Further away, I can see two lit circles with witches, and Merlin with a baby in his arms. And in the distance, Quakers of all kinds, along with a lookalike Dr. Mengele and Karl Brandt walking round and round.

Round and round.

Above, drones and dragons of the Apocalypse turning and turning.

Wrooom, wroooom.

Wroooom, wrooooom.

Wroooom, wrooooom.

Further afield, the *ankou* is there with his cart, waiting.

Then, I can see him, far away, in the distance.

I do not know who I am, yet I feel alive, I am not scared.

In one movement, I take my kithara and walk down the hill, diagonally, through the crowd. Nobody is looking at me.

I am invisible, I am anonymous. Yet, I feel in full bloom, my porcelain skin with green stripes of moss and soil, my golden blonde curls balancing freely with entangled sweet chestnut leaves, my umbilicus already healed and pierced with a green emerald gem, my breast full and high, my long legs happy to walk, my bare feet feeling the earth and my womb ready to receive the chosen seed.

With an intense, dreamy feeling of *omoiyari*, I walk endlessly towards him in the ever-expanding yet ephemeral world of my dream.

Love Your Book

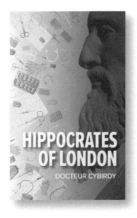

Hippocrates of London

TIMELINE

OCTOBER 2022

Soft-back book printed from paper that has been carbon offset through the World Land Trust Scheme.

PRINTED by Swallowtail Print
at Norwich, Norfolk, United Kingdom

PUBLISHED by Cybirdy Publishing
London, United Kingdom

CYBIRDY
Publishing Limited

SPECIAL EDITION
Autographed by the Author

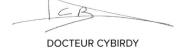

DOCTEUR CYBIRDY

Cherish your book

WHO are you?	WHO did you obtain the book from?	WHEN did you obtain the book
FIRST GUARDIAN		
SECOND GUARDIAN		
THIRD GUARDIAN		
FOURTH GUARDIAN		
FIFTH GUARDIAN		

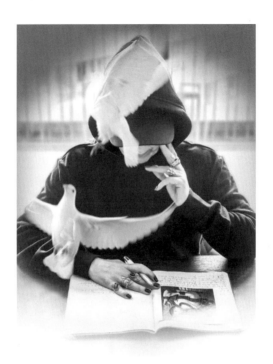

Docteur Cybirdy is a faceless writer and a General Physician who has practiced medicine for the past thirty years in France and in the UK. She graduated first in France as a General Physician specialised in tropical diseases, and then studied epidemiology, public health and nutrition at the London School of Hygiene and Tropical Medicine.

For the past twenty-three years, Docteur Cybirdy has been an independent medical doctor in London. In the pre-Covid era, and in the midst of political debates on euthanasia and abortion, the doctor felt the need to write and tell.

Passionate about art of medicine and ethics, in *Hippocrates of London*, her debut novel, she shares her anecdotes with humanity and dignity, with a literary twist removed from hyper-rationality.